DANCE!

Therapy for Dancers

DANCE!

Therapy for Dancers

BERYL DUNN M.C.S.P.

PHYSIOTHERAPIST TO THE ROYAL BALLET COMPANY, LONDON

INTRODUCTION BY DAME MARGOT FONTEYN

FOREWORD BY H. JACKSON BURROWS

Photographs by Philip Raymond-Barker

HEINEMANN HEALTH BOOKS

LONDON

First published 1974
Reprinted 1979

ISBN 0 433 07960 6

Filmset and printed by BAS Printers Limited, Over Wallop, Hampshire

IN

MEMORY

OF

IVOR ROBERTSON

CONSULTANT ORTHOPAEDIC SURGEON

TO THE

ROYAL BALLET COMPANY

1959–1972

The author would like to thank dancers of the Royal Ballet Company for their co-operation and in particular Deirdre O'Conaire for her technical advice

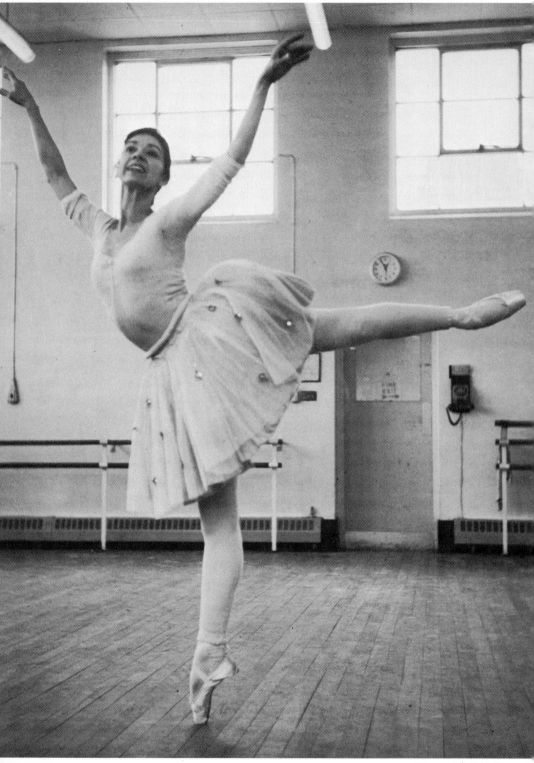

Photograph by Keith Money

INTRODUCTION by

DAME MARGOT FONTEYN

The technique of classical ballet is designed in such a way that dancers who execute it perfectly should never suffer injury. But since the necessary physical perfection rarely exists it is an advantage for us to understand how best to deal with our limitations.

Beryl Dunn gives us the knowledge she has accumulated over 14 years of treating the Royal Ballet Company. During this time her day to day concentration on the special ills of ballet dancers must be unique in the world.

She presents this knowledge clearly and simply; so all of us, teachers, students and dancers of ballet and modern dancing will want to study this book and profit by her wise words.

Margot Fonteyn Arias

FOREWORD by

H. JACKSON BURROWS, C.B.E., F.R.C.S.

*Honorary Consulting Orthopaedic Surgeon St Bartholomews Hospital and
Royal National Orthopaedic Hospital*

Miss Dunn has set out to diminish the risk of injury to ballet dancers and to help those called upon to treat them. Rather than approach her subject from a detailed consideration of ballet technique or of anatomy, she gives an outline in simple terms of the positions and movements of classical ballet, the strains they impose on persons of differing physique and how the effects of these can be met. In doing so, she is an artist in reducing jargon—the terminology of a discipline—to simple everyday terms. Few could do this so well.

Her descriptions are those of a chartered physiotherapist who rightly has gained and retained the confidence of members of the Royal Ballet by her personality and expertise. Fourteen years as its "resident" physiotherapist have given her an almost unrivalled experience. The fruits of this she hands on. The methods she describes are those that she, personally, has found to work.

It may well be asked "why all this fuss about ballet injuries; do they differ from other injuries?" The answer is that they do not differ fundamentally from other closed injuries, but they do often differ in the precise mechanism of infliction, in the particular form that they take and in their relative incidence. Some generalizations should make this clear. Ballet requires of its participants not only qualities of personality and morale—discipline, devotion, gregariousness, imperturbability, adaptability, endurance and infinite capacity for hard work—but also special qualities of physique. These are partly endowed and partly attained by arduous training from an early age at which the growing and developing body can be moulded to achieve postures and movements far outside the range of ordinary human ability. In other words ballet, though an art, demands the agility and strength of a specially trained contortionist. By skill and grace these are transmuted into a beautiful and entrancing art. Great stresses are often imposed under quite unusual mechanical conditions. These vary with different physiques; for a simple instance, the ballet dancer whose legs cannot be turned out adequately at the hips may, in attempting to compensate, strain knees and feet, and this may be worsened by bad training. Selection of children of unsuitable physique can be the basic fault, but children's development cannot be fully foreseen.

Just as there is nothing fundamentally distinct in the nature of ballet injuries, so also treatment does not depart from fundamental principles. An acute injury requires initial rest in its several forms and, at the proper time, exercise. The circumstances of ballet naturally encourage attempted short cuts, which must be resisted. For instance, injecting an injured joint with an anti-inflammatory substance may allow early use by abolishing the warnings of pain and restrictive muscle spasm, but only to the detriment of the joint: a sacrifice of the future to the present.

There is much more that could be said about ballet as a different world. The important point here is that the differences are enough to make the observations and experience of a dedicated physiotherapist well worth recording and well worth studying. We are grateful to Miss Dunn.

CONTENTS

		Page No.
	Introduction	vii
	Foreword	ix
	Author's Introduction	xiii
1	Principal Positions of Classical Ballet	1
2	Anatomy	13
3	Posture	20
4	Muscle Tone	27
5	Relaxation	29
6	Breathing Exercises	31
7	Variations in Physique	33
8	Hints on Injury Prevention	52
9	General Health	55
10	Non-Weight-Bearing Exercises	58
11	Treatment	64
	Glossary—Ballet Terms	92
	Glossary—Medical Terms	93
	Summary	95
	Index	96

AUTHOR'S INTRODUCTION

This book is dedicated, not to the few dancers with perfect physique, but to the many dancers who are struggling to express their art with a less-than-perfect instrument.

They have to learn to understand their bodies and live with their limitations, adapting them to the demands of ballet in the best way possible.

Except in the last chapter describing common injuries, no medical terms are used, and advice is based on visual perception, which is so well developed in dancers.

Chapter *I*

Principal Positions of
Classical Ballet

This first chapter shows the principal positions of classical ballet as demonstrated by Merle Park and Anthony Dowell.

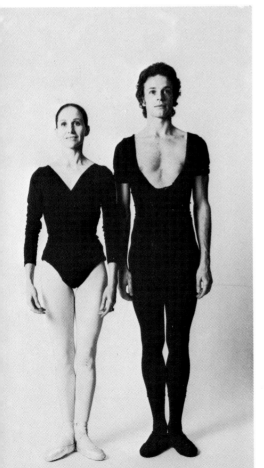

1. Male and female dancers
This is an example of a perfect male and female physique.

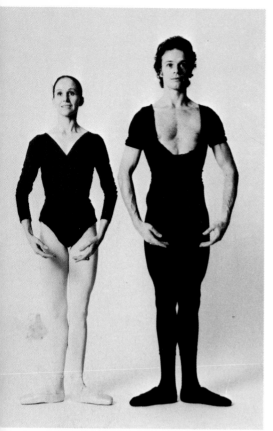

2. 1st position
The feet are rotated out to 180°. The heels are together and the knees are straight. The whole body is pulled up, making the dancers as tall as possible.

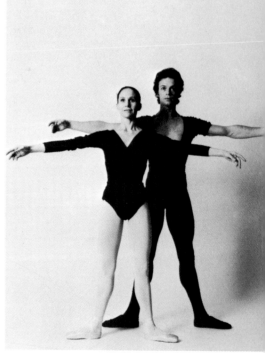

3. 2nd position
The feet are turned out to 180° as in 1st position. The distance between the heels should be one and a half times the length of the dancer's own foot.

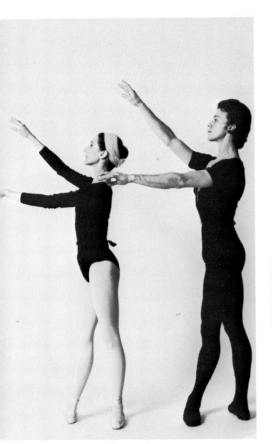

4. 4th position (in profile)
The feet are turned out to 180° as in 1st position with one foot placed in front of the other leaving a gap between the feet.

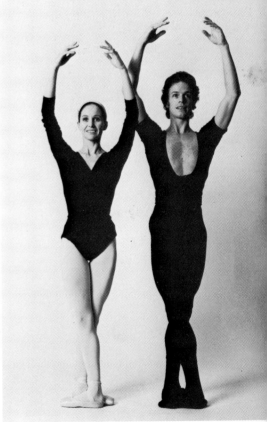

5. 5th position
With the feet turned out to 180° one foot is placed directly in front of the other. The knees are pulled up and quite straight.

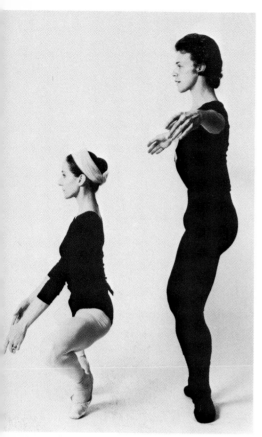

6. Demi and full plié in 1st position

Demi plié is bending the knees to the fullest extent without raising the heels. Full *plié* is bending the knees fully allowing the heels to rise. In both cases the back is held straight and vertical.

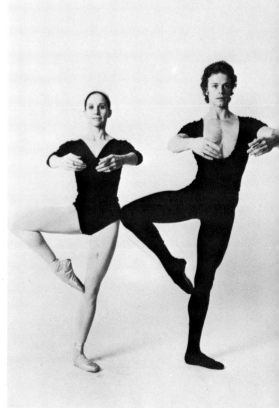

7. Retiré

The supporting leg is turned out to $180°$. The working leg is also fully turned out and the hip is flexed to $90°$ so that the pointed foot touches the supporting knee.

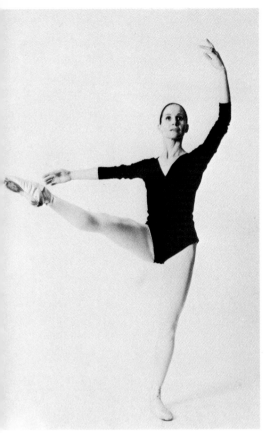

8. Effacé devant
The dancer stands on one leg with the other leg raised forward in an "open" position. Note the lack of tension in the upper part of the body.

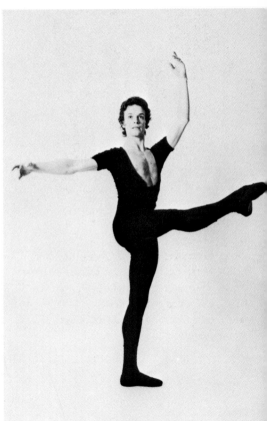

9. Croisé devant
The dancer stands on one leg with the other leg raised forwards in a "crossed" position.

10. A la seconde

Here the dancer stands on one leg with the other leg raised to the side.

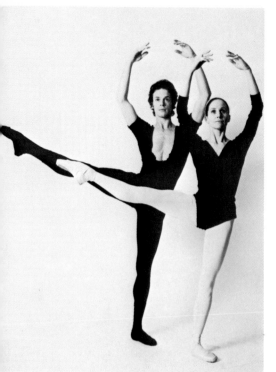

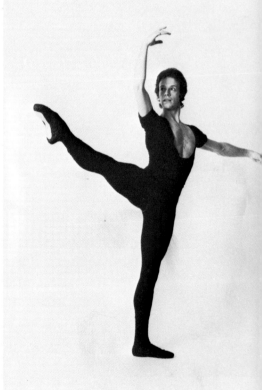

11. Ecarté devant

The dancer is in an *à la seconde* position facing diagonally forwards with the head turned towards the raised leg.

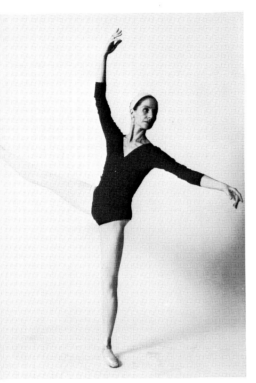

12. Ecarté derrière
The dancer is in an *à la seconde* position facing diagonally backwards with the head turned away from the raised leg.

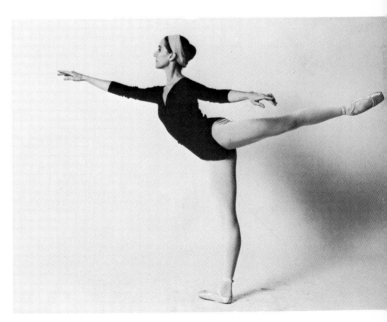

13. 1st arabesque
The dancer stands on one leg with the other leg raised directly behind in an "open" position.

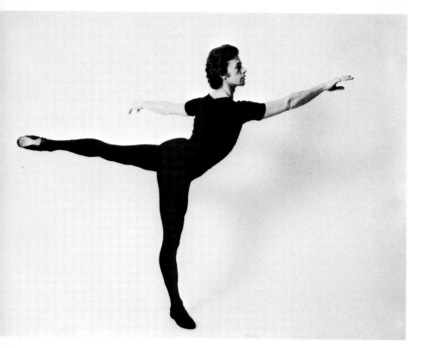

14. Epaulé arabesque
The dancer stands on one leg with
the other leg raised directly behind in
a "crossed" position.

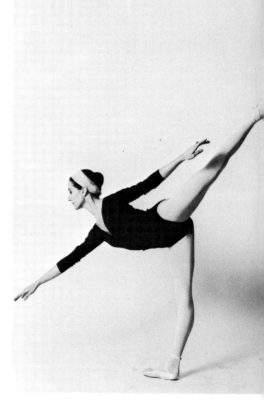

15. Arabesque penchée
This is one of the loveliest positions
in classical ballet. The dancer stands
on one leg and lifts the other leg as
high as possible at the back allowing
the body to tip forward on the supporting leg. Note the continuing
line between the front arm and the
back leg.

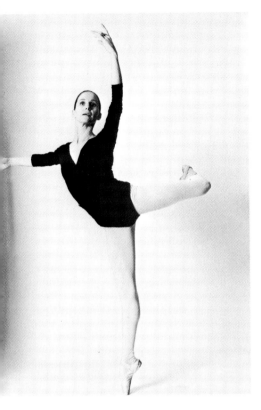

16. Attitude effacé on point

The dancer stands on one leg on point and the other leg is lifted behind with the knee flexed to 90°.

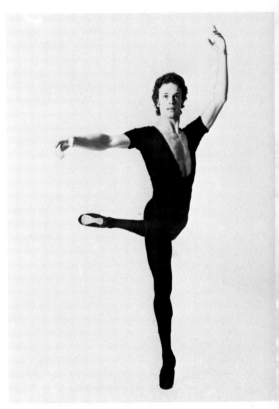

17. Attitude croisé on half point

The dancer stands on one leg on demi-point and the other leg is lifted behind with the knee flexed to 90°.

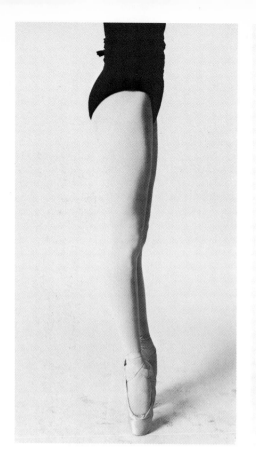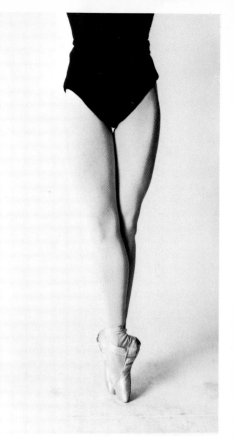

18 and 19. On point in 1st and 5th position

The photographs demonstrate the leg perfectly pulled up on point.

20–23. Correct lifting ▶

Note how in each photograph the man's back is pulled up maintaining the normal curves of the spine. The curves should not increase under the extra weight. (Contrast Figs. 88–90, page 53)

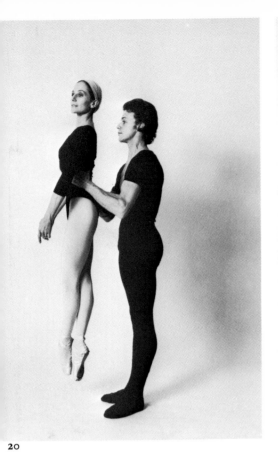

20

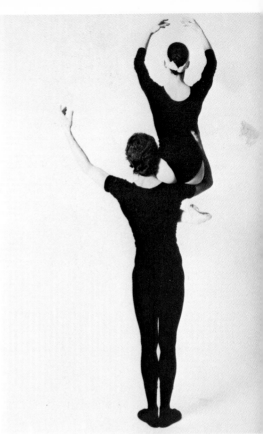

21

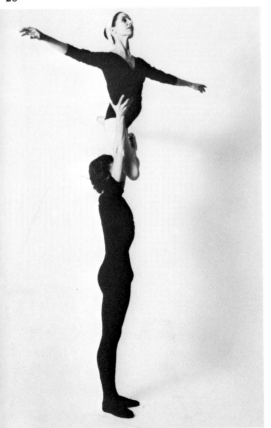

22

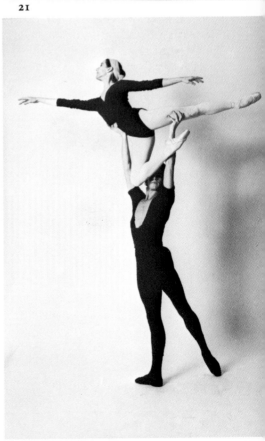

23

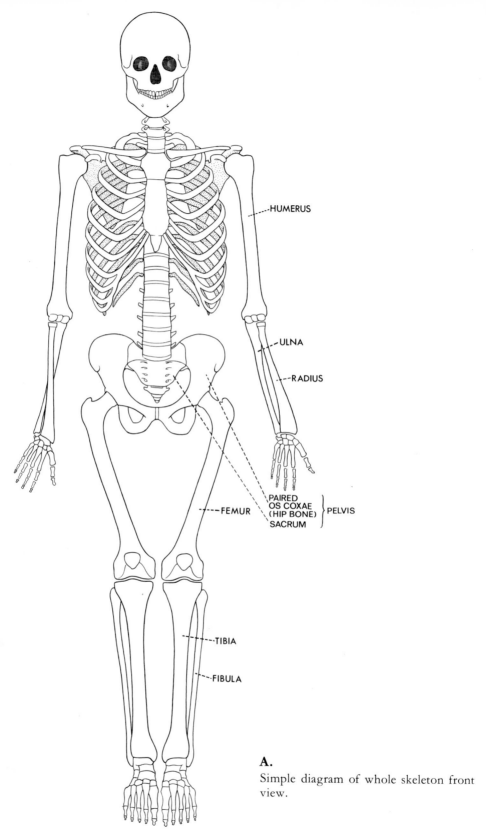

HUMERUS

ULNA

RADIUS

FEMUR

PAIRED
OS COXAE
(HIP BONE)   } PELVIS
SACRUM

TIBIA

FIBULA

A.
Simple diagram of whole skeleton front view.

Chapter *2*

Anatomy

Without going into anatomical detail I would like in this chapter to explain the basic structure of the body and how different types of movement take place in different joints. (Diagram A. Whole skeleton).

Dancers think only of the shape that they can make with their bodies, but if they could learn to isolate and move each joint in turn they would understand that a given shape is the summation of movements in a number of joints.

The unique factor in ballet compared with other athletic activities is the extreme range of movement required in each joint. In this context both dancer and therapist should be very aware that, after a joint or muscle injury, the first aim should be to restore full movement, because a stiff joint will diminish the art of a dancer.

A JOINT—is a meeting point between two bones which are held together by bands of strong fibrous material called ligaments and by muscles. Where the bones come in contact they are covered with a smooth glistening substance called "articular cartilage". The movement in any particular joint should not force the ends of the bones beyond the limit of this articular cartilage (Diagram B).

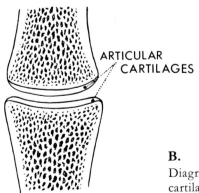

ARTICULAR
CARTILAGES

B.
Diagram of joint showing articular cartilage.

The danger of forcing too much movement in any one joint is to predispose that joint towards early wear and tear in later life.

There are several types of joints in the body and each type allows different movement, e.g.

1. Hinge Joint—the ankle is an example of a hinge joint, allowing movement in one plane. The knee is principally a hinge joint, but once the knee is bent even a few degrees it does allow some rotation.
2. Ball and Socket Joint—the shoulder and hip are examples of this type of joint and allow movement in all three planes.
3. Gliding Joints—where one bone glides on another allowing a small amount of movement, e.g. in the small bones of the foot in front of the ankle joint.

THE SPINE—The spinal column is made up of a series of small bones (vertebrae) held together by muscles and ligaments and separated by small pads called

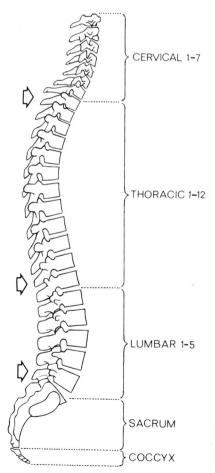

CERVICAL 1–7

THORACIC 1–12

LUMBAR 1–5

SACRUM

COCCYX

C.
Diagram of spine sideview. Arrows mark vulnerable areas where curves join.

intervertebral discs. Each vertebra comprises a solid body in front which carries the weight and an arch behind which transmits the spinal cord and nerves and provides an anchorage for spinal muscles. The discs make up a quarter of the length of the spine and they act as shock absorbers. They vary in shape and thickness and so help to form the natural curves of the spine (Diagram C).

There are three main natural curves in the spine:

1. The neck with its seven cervical vertebrae curves forward;
2. The chest with its 12 thoracic vertebrae curves backward;
3. The five lumbar vertebrae form the hollow of the back and curve forwards.

These curves, as seen in the diagram of the spine, with the aid of the intervertebral discs, greatly enhance the ability of the spine to absorb shock.

The solid bottom part of the spine consists of five sacral vertebrae fused together and of a small "tail" at the end of the spine called the coccyx.

Any permanent alteration in one curve will affect the curve above or below it, e.g. an increased lumbar curve or hollow back results in an increased thoracic curve or round back and then probably an increased cervical curve with a poking head, which is particularly ugly (Figs. 24, 25).

24. Bad posture with increased spinal curves.

25. Good posture.

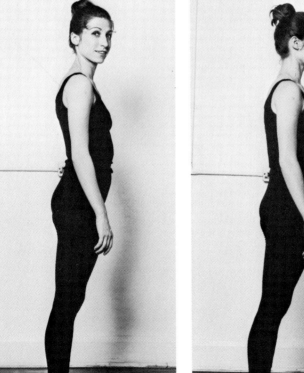

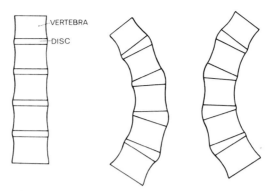

D.
Diagram of the flexibility of the spine allowed by the discs.

The movement in each joint of the spine is quite small and is produced by compression of the disc in different directions (Diagram D).

In order to get maximum movement in the spine each joint must work fully, BUT if too much movement is expected at one level there is over-compression of the disc at this level, leading to damage and pain.

The particularly vulnerable parts of the spine are those where one curve joins the next, i.e. the bottom of the neck, the bottom of the chest, and the bottom of the back where it joins the solid pelvis (Diagram C, arrows indicate vulnerable parts).

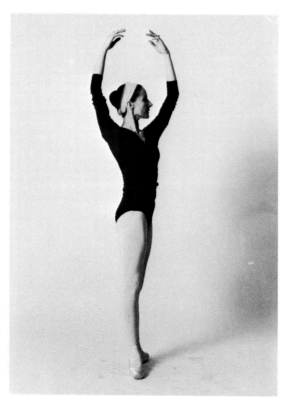

26. Rotation in the thoracic spine.

Different parts of the spine specialise in different types of movement:

1. The Cervical or Neck Region allows movement in all directions. To feel this yourself, sit with your shoulders quite relaxed and still, move your head forwards, backwards, from side to side, and then turn round to look over each shoulder.

2. The Thoracic or Chest Region—Because of the attachment of the rib cage in this area movement backwards and sideways is limited, BUT this area specialises in rotation. To feel this rotation stand in the 1st position and keep your pelvis facing forwards. Now turn your shoulders to look behind you and feel where the movement takes place (Fig. 26).

It should be noted here that the other place where rotation occurs is in the hip joints. It is quite possible to stand and look behind by rotating on the hip joints

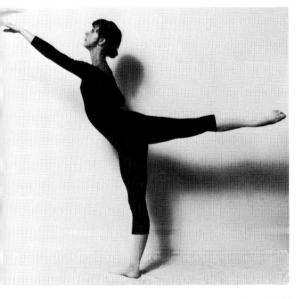

27. Good *arabesque.*

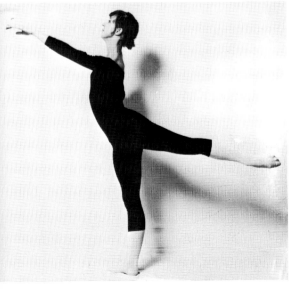

28. Bad *arabesque.*

without using the thoracic spine. This is a particular problem in ballet because so much emphasis has to be put on the strong control of the shoulders over the hips in order to do pirouettes etc., that sometimes the muscles controlling free rotation in the thoracic spine are neglected.

3. Lumbar Region—The five lumbar vertebrae are the biggest and strongest in the spine. They allow movement forwards, backwards, and sideways, but only very limited rotation.

4. The Sacrum—This is the solid base of the spine and forms part of the pelvis (Diagram A page 12). The joints joining it to the rest of the pelvis (i.e. to the hip bones) are the paired sacro-iliac joints. The joint between the fifth lumbar vertebra and the sacrum is known as the lumbo-sacral joint—it is very vulnerable to over-use during back extension. (Fig. 27 showing a correct *arabesque* with back extension shared between all the joints of the spine and Fig. 28 showing an incorrect *arabesque* with hyper-extension or too much movement at lumbo-sacral joint.)

The best exercise I know to encourage extension in the whole spine and not just at the bottom of the back is as follows:

Exercise to develop mobility in upper spine.

| 29 | 30 | 31 |

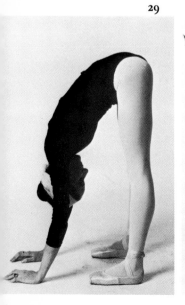 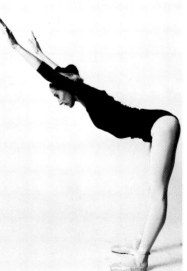 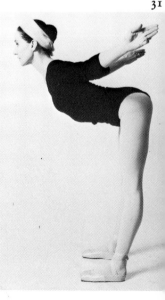

1. Stand with the feet apart and bend forward so that the hands touch the floor.
2. Straighten the back, arching the upper part as much as possible, but without letting the lower back lift more than 90° from the legs.
3. Drop the head and shoulders loosely towards the floor again and repeat several times before straightening up. The arms can either turn out at the sides of the body or swing up above the head (Figs. 29, 30, 31).

Flexion or forward bending of the spine is something that should be practised daily, especially by dancers with long hamstring muscles (the muscles at the back of the thighs).

To do this, stand up straight, let the head drop forward, and then allow each joint to bend in turn until the hands reach the floor, then straighten up in the same way. It is very easy for a dancer with long hamstrings to jack-knife forwards on the hip joints, keeping the back quite stiff. This may result eventually in a stiff back which also means a comparatively weak and much less beautiful back (Figs. 32, 33).

Jack-knife.

32

Back flexion.

33

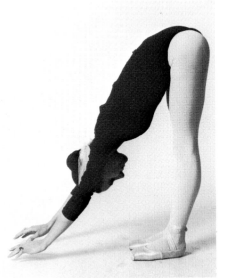
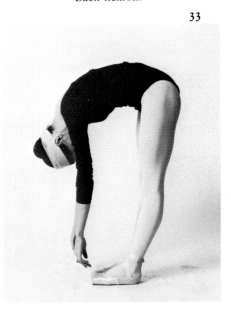

Chapter *3*

Posture

Developing a good posture means training the nervous impulses or reflexes from the muscles so that they automatically maintain enough "tone" to balance each other and so produce not only the most perfect positions visually, but the most economical positions from which the body can perform. This postural training cannot be over emphasised because it concerns the basic body placement. Once good posture is learnt, the dancer can assume a correct posture without looking into the mirror, because the correct "feeling" is felt from within the muscles. All developing movements of the arms and legs are then performed on a correct base. There is no doubt that only with the most perfect and economical use of the body can the very demanding rôles in ballet be performed. If movements stem from faulty posture, a dancer's technique is like a house with poor foundations, and sooner or later, if the more difficult rôles in ballet are tackled, the basic placement will have to be re-learnt correctly.

Teaching of Correct Posture

The first thing to learn is control of the pelvis, which is the link between the body and the legs.

1. The dancer should stand by the barre with the feet turned out making no more than $90°$ between them. She should then practise sticking her bottom out and then tucking it in.
    NO MOVEMENT SHOULD TAKE PLACE ABOVE THE WAIST. This tipping of the pelvis forwards and backwards takes place at the lumbo-sacral joint by alternate contraction of the abdominal muscles and the bottom muscles.
2. Having become aware of this pelvic movement below the waist, the dancer should then once more stick her bottom out, then she should tuck her bottom in, but only so far; there should still be a *slight* forward curve in the lower spine.
3. Holding the pelvis quite steady, the dancer should then pull up her knee muscles, and lift the weight of the body upwards so that she feels as tall

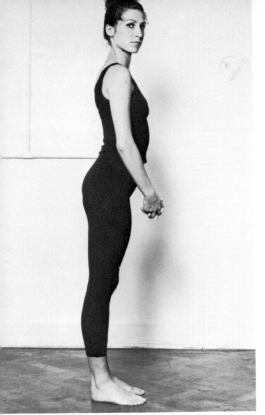
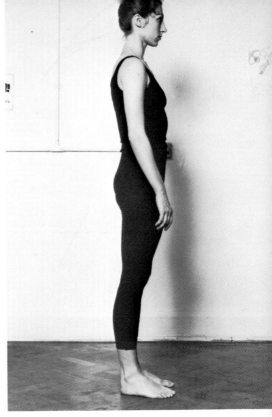

34. "Bottom out."

35. "Bottom in," weight on heels.

Posture correction.

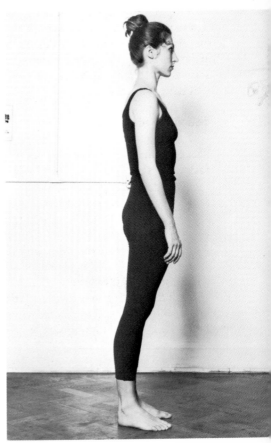

36. Line of weight falling through balls of feet. Correct.

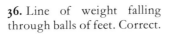

and weightless as possible. The shoulders should retract slightly, opening up the front of the chest; the chin should be in; and the crown of the head should be uppermost.

4. If the lower rib cage sticks out, a small contraction of the abdominal muscles will bring the lower rib cage and the front pelvic bones closer together to correct this.

5. The head and shoulders having been positioned correctly over the pelvis the weight should then be transferred from the heels to the balls of the feet: this is done at the ANKLE JOINT (Figs. 34, 35, 36).

This exercise should be repeated again and again until the correct position is achieved automatically. Only then should the feet be moved to first position. Forward transfer of weight becomes much more difficult in this position as it can only be done across the width of the foot instead of from heel to toe and is, therefore, across a much smaller base. BUT the transference of weight must take place in the foot and not, as is so often the case, by letting the pelvis come forward and leaving the body above the waist tipped slightly backwards (Figs. 37, 38, 39).

There is a danger of tucking the bottom in too far or over-correcting the pelvic tilt. By so doing, the natural curves are diminished too much, making the spine too rigid and less able to absorb shock, especially when jumping. Sometimes the bottom is tucked in so much that the lumbar spine curves backwards. This habit, once established, will make the lower back much more injury-prone (Fig. 40).

▶

Posture correction in 1st position.
37. "Bottom out"
38. "Bottom in"
39. Correct.
40. Over-correction of pelvic tilt.

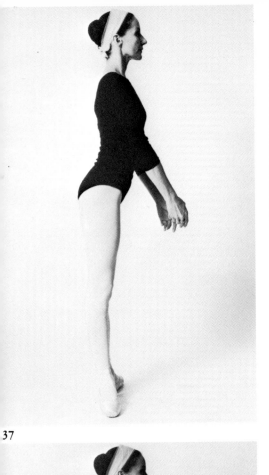

37

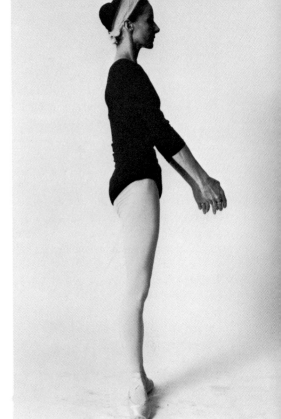

38

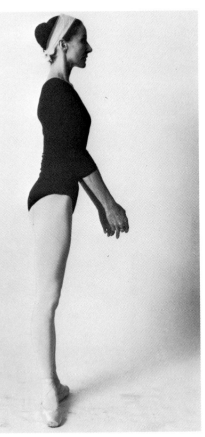

39

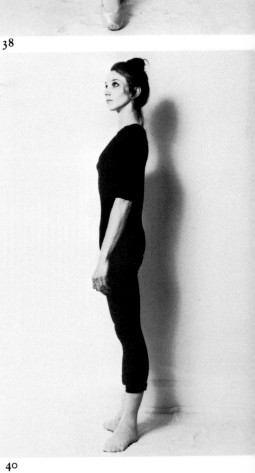

40

The Poking Head

This is very unsightly and greatly detracts from the presence of a dancer (Fig. 41). Correction depends on learning to shift the head and shoulders back on the shoulder girdle AND NOT on the waist.

It will be seen that in Fig. 43 the line of weight remains correctly on the balls of the feet, but in Fig. 42 it is shifted back to the heels.

The following exercise is very useful in training for correct holding of the head:

1. Stand with the feet apart; and drop the body loosely forward so that the hands touch the floor;

2. Extend the back until it becomes horizontal. Feel a straight line from the back of the head to the bottom—the arms should be by the sides, the chin in, and the head and neck shifted back. In this position movement of the head and shoulders backwards will be felt between the shoulder blades and NOT at the waist.

3. Relax with the hands to the floor again. Repeat several times (Fig. 44).

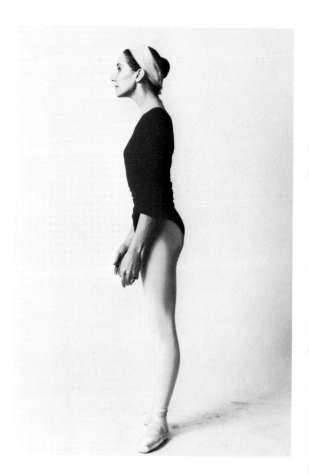

41. Poking head.

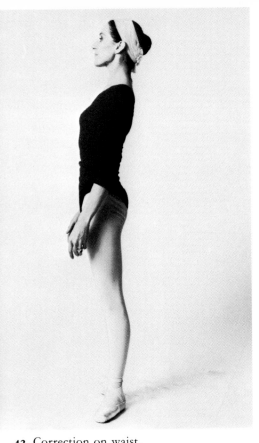

42. Correction on waist.

43. Correction on shoulder girdle.

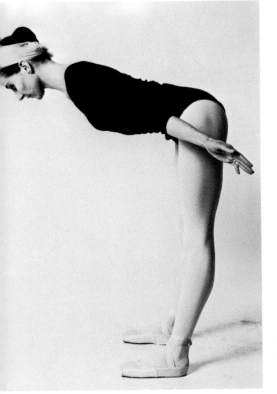

44. Exercise to teach correct positioning of the head.

To recapitulate on posture training :

1. The spinal curves are pulled up but not obliterated.
2. The head and neck are retracted on the shoulder girdle and not on the waist.
3. The abdominal muscles are kept slightly contracted to stop the lower ribs sticking out.
4. The knee muscles are pulled up but the knees are not snapped back.
5. The line of weight is shifted forward so that it falls through the big toe joints.

Chapter 4

Muscle Tone

Muscle tone accounts for the "feel" of a muscle during rest. It can be increased by general health and fitness but the variation from "high" to "low" tone in different individuals is something personal.

High Tone

People who have high tone in their muscles are usually strong. The muscles feel hard even when at rest and there is less slack to be taken up in the muscles when they contract. These dancers can get fit in a much shorter time after a spell off, BUT the problem for these dancers is to make their muscles relax enough to keep the blood circulating freely, especially in quick movements. Often with this type of body the joints are not so free and the dancer has a constant struggle for mobility. (See chapter on Relaxation). One very famous character dancer in the Royal Ballet had such "high" tone in his muscles he found that if he did class every day he became so muscle-bound he could hardly move at all!

Low Tone

This produces muscles that are floppy and soft to feel and are usually associated with loose joints. This type of body is often beautiful in the shapes it can make but is very difficult to control. There is much slack to take up when the muscles contract; furthermore, if there are loose joints, the muscles have to work extra hard to hold the joints correctly.

The training of these dancers when young requires infinite time and trouble, and fatigue must be avoided at all costs. A little work done correctly is much more important than a long period when fatigue sets in and bad habits develop. It takes longer for these dancers to get fit after a rest and they get unfit much more quickly during a period of inactivity. They also tire more easily because all the time they are having to work harder than their opposites.

These descriptions of people with "High" and "Low" tone in their muscles are, of course, extreme cases—the majority fall somewhere in the middle. For the extreme cases their problems are so different that one wonders if they should be taught in separate classes. In the one group there is the problem of keeping the muscles relaxed and at the same time trying to increase mobility in the joints; and in the other group the problem of controlling over-mobile joints.

Chapter *5*

Relaxation

The greater the demands on the body, the more important the art of relaxation becomes. It should be taught from the beginning of ballet training and the dancer should be so aware of tension that she can relax a muscle in the same way in which she can contract it.

By avoiding unnecessary tension the blood-flow through working muscles can be increased and fatigue decreased. When a muscle relaxes from prolonged tension, the blood-flow through it increases many times, bringing food to the muscle and taking away waste products.

Dame Margot Fonteyn once said to me at an age when most dancers have long since retired, "I can no longer spare the energy to be nervous." "Nerves" produce tension which wastes energy.

Except for jumping, which requires a maximum of effort from all resources, all positions should be held and all movements performed with the minimum of muscle action. How often one sees dancers pulling up the thighs, pointing the toes, or lifting the arms with far more muscle exertion than is needed to produce the movement or hold the position. This does not mean, for example, that the thighs should not be pulled up fully, but it does mean that enough muscle action should be used and NO MORE.

A good exercise for detecting shoulder tension is first to shrug your shoulders to your ears and then let them relax so that you feel the difference between tension and relaxation. Then lift your arm to $90°$ and support it at this level. Let the shoulder muscles relax so that the arm is quite supported, and then lift the arm off the support with the minimum of muscle necessary (Figs. 45, 46).

Practising the Art of Relaxation

There is a record called "How to Relax in Body and in Mind" by Margaret Smith, M.C.S.P., which can be obtained from Recorded Sound Ltd., 27-31 Bryanston Street, London, W.1. This is well worth having. First, it instructs you to lie flat and then to concentrate on each joint as the muscles around it are made to contract and then relax. After a time you will become aware of the feeling of relaxation.

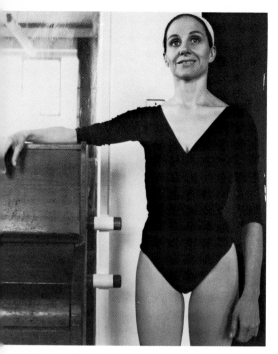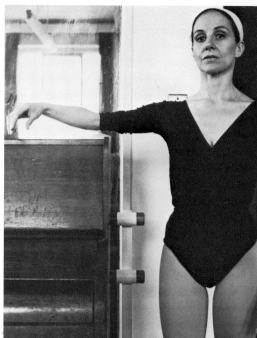

45 and **46.** Exercise to reduce shoulder tension.

The next stage is to take each position at the barre and to make sure before beginning an exercise that no unnecessary muscle fibres are being used to hold the position.

The third stage is to keep thinking during the exercise whether there is unnecessary tension in the body. Even during sustained exercises it is important to find momentary relaxation between movements. Sustained exercises on one leg with no relaxation produce tension and aching as the muscles struggle to work without a proper blood-flow.

Chapter *6*

Breathing Exercises

These are valuable because they help to develop lung expansion and thereby increase the oxygen intake to the body. Also, performed rhythmically, they are a great antidote to tension. When practising breathing exercises lie flat on your back with your knees bent and NEVER take more than three to four deep breaths at a time. Air should be taken in through the nose and blown out through the mouth. Particular attention should be paid to lung expansion in three areas of the chest.

1. *Apical Breathing*—this is expansion at the top of the lungs under the collar bones. Put one hand flat over each collar bone, and, as you breathe in, concentrate on pushing the hands up as the lungs expand and, as you breathe out, let the hands press gently down on the top of the rib cage. While doing this the sides of the ribs and tummy should remain as still

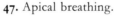

47. Apical breathing.

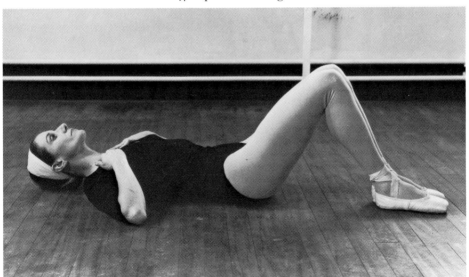

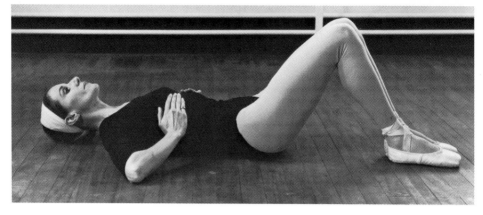

48. Lateral breathing.

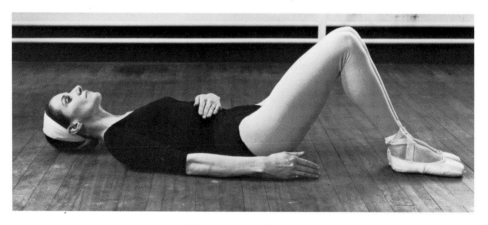

49. Diaphragmatic breathing.

as possible. This area is often neglected in dancers because of tension in the muscles of the shoulder girdle (Fig 47).

2. *Lateral Breathing*—this is the expansion of the lower part of the lungs sideways. Put your hands on either side of the chest wall. Breathe in and let the lung expansion push the hands out sideways; breathe out giving gentle pressure on the ribs to aid expulsion of the air. While doing this try to keep the top of the chest and the tummy quite still and just concentrate on the lungs expanding sideways (Fig. 48).

3. *Diaphragmatic or Abdominal Breathing*—to practise this the chest wall should remain quite still and relaxed. Place one hand on the top of the abdomen where the ribs divide. As the air is taken in, the top of the stomach rises, taking the hand with it, and then descends as the air is expelled (Fig. 49).

The Over-developed Diaphragm—This is not uncommon in dancers and comes from over-emphasis on abdominal breathing. It is very often associated with tension round the neck and shoulder causing neglect of the upper part of the lungs and over-use of the diaphragm.

Chapter 7

Variations in Physique

The perfect physique is the exception and not the rule. Most dancers have some problem that they have to live with and adapt in the best way possible to the demands of ballet.

It has been my practice with the Royal Ballet Company to chart the range of movement in joints and to note the variation from one side of the body to the other (See chart on page 69). In this way a dancer can be made aware of his or her problems and often helped to prevent the common injuries that are related to certain physiques.

Some problems in physique are a direct result of inadequate supervision during early training. It is very important with a growing child that ligaments in weight-bearing joints should not be allowed to stretch where they affect the

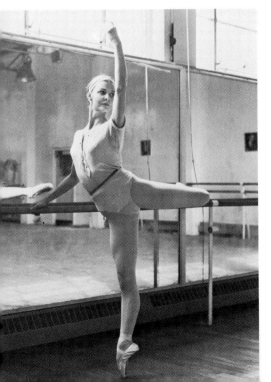

50. Note the straight line at the knee and ankle which denotes strength.

strength and line of the dancer, because, once stretched, they are stretched for life and will cause permanent weakness in the dancer's physique.

Sway-back Knees (over-extended)

To check for sway-back knees and to compare one knee with the other sit with the knees out straight. Pull up the knee muscles so that the knees are pressed back and the feet lift off the floor. If one foot lifts higher than the other it is because there is more movement backwards at the corresponding knee joint (Fig. 51). Even a small variation will affect the whole line of weight through the leg.

One of the causes of sway-back knees is pressing the knees back instead of pulling up when they are straightened. When a child is growing and the ligaments are soft, snapping the knees back may gradually stretch the ligaments at the back of the knee. If this is seen to be happening, the child should be watched very carefully and made to pull up the thigh muscles, keeping the knee firm but not pressed back. On no account should the child be allowed to tire as this is one cause of snapping the knees back. When working in 1st position the heels should be kept together so that the knees are supported against each other (Figs. 52, 53).

Another cause of sway-back knees is stretching the muscles at the back of the thighs (hamstrings) with just the foot supported on the barre. If the knee is showing any sign of becoming over-extended, it is much wiser to support the whole leg, before leaning over to stretch the back of the thigh (Figs. 54, 55).

It is not easy to overcome the problem of sway-back knees but I have known several principal dancers of the Royal Ballet who have done so. The difficulty is in

51. Test for "sway-back" knees.

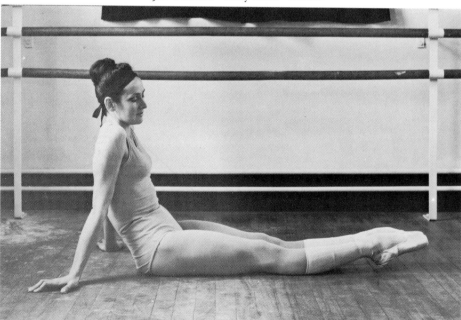

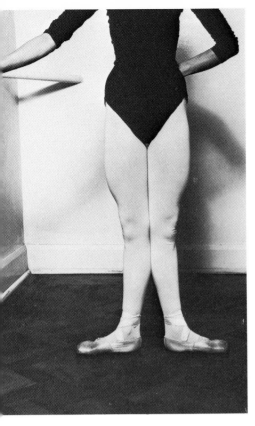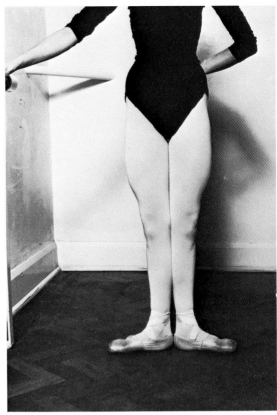

52. Incorrect.

53. Correct.

54. Foot supported.

Hamstring stretch

55. Leg supported.

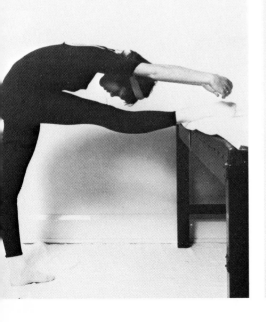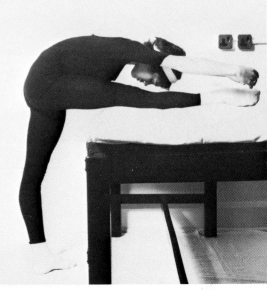

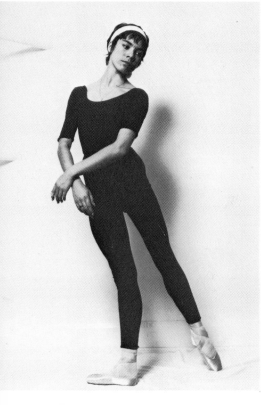
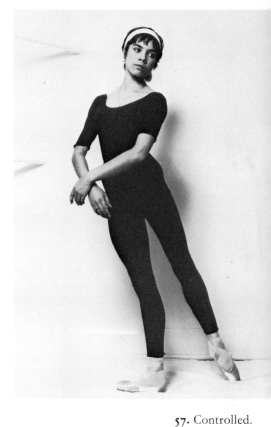

56. Uncontrolled.

57. Controlled.

Sway-back knees

58. Uncontrolled.

59. Controlled.

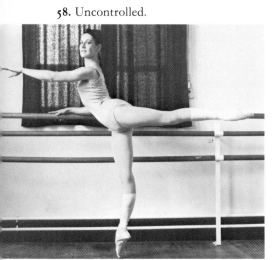
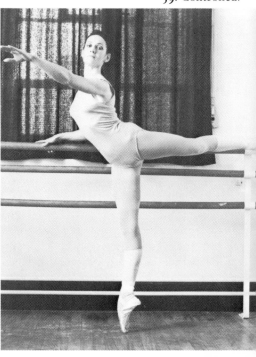

shifting the line of weight forward over the balls of the feet. Besides transferring the weight forward at the ankle joints, there has to be a slight shift of the pelvis forward on the hip joints, and very firm muscular control of the knee joints. Individual help should be sought with this problem (Figs. 56, 57, 58, 59).

Lower-Leg Rotation

It is not uncommon to find undue rotation of the lower leg taking place at the knee joint, especially with dancers whose hips have a poor turn-out. This comes from forcing the feet out beyond the line of the knee and hip in the young dancer. To check this, sit with your knees straight and the knee-cap facing the ceiling, then pull up the ankle joint so that the toes come towards the knee and see if the feet

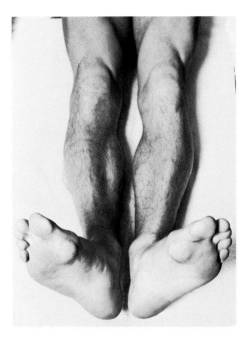

60. Outward rotation of the lower leg.

are in line with the knee-cap. If not, see how much rotation there is in the lower leg. Once rotation has occurred the knees can never come correctly over the ankle joint in a *plié* and the correct line of weight has been lost (Fig. 60).

As has already been stated, the knee is principally a hinge joint allowing movement in one plane. However, when the knee is bent even a few degrees, it does allow a certain amount of rotation. The less rotational strain put on the knee joint the better. When standing in ballet positions with the knees straight, and especially when standing on one leg, it is very important to keep the knee muscles really pulled up so as not to allow even a little bend at the knee joint. Only when the knee joint is fully extended does it allow no rotation; so it is only in this position that it is really stable and protected from injury.

Feet

Another common place for stretching ligaments is along the inner border of the foot. If the feet are turned out beyond the line of the knee and hip, and if the arches in the foot are not held correctly, then the foot rolls in. The inner border of the foot bulges and its ligaments may become irreversibly stretched. When young and strong, a flattened arch may cause no trouble. Later, however, the foot will become more accident prone (Fig. 61).

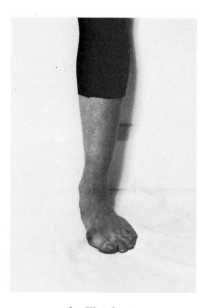

61. Flat foot.

Turn-out (outward rotation) at the Hips

Dancers will be all too aware whether they have a good turn-out or not, but it is worth lying in a "frog" position (Figs. 62, 63) and noticing if there is the same amount of turn-out in both hips. If one hip is more restricted, allowance should be made for this fact; otherwise if the feet are turned out an equal amount, the strain will fall on the inner side of the knee or ankle.

Outward rotation of the hips is the most unusual position of balletic movement, and three main groups of muscles are used to this end. The most important are, of course, the deep muscles at the back of the hip joints which not only turn the hips out to their maximum but hold them in this position throughout each exercise. (See Exercise 1.)

At the same time the muscles on the inner side of the thigh should contract, thus helping to rotate the thigh bones. (See Exercise 2.)

With the hips thus held in the best position the joints will allow, the line of weight should run straight through the knee joints and the ankle joints and the feet should be placed on the floor in line with the ankle and knee. Even so, the untrained or weak foot will tend to roll in and this should be controlled by the small muscles in the feet. (See Exercise 3.)

Frog position

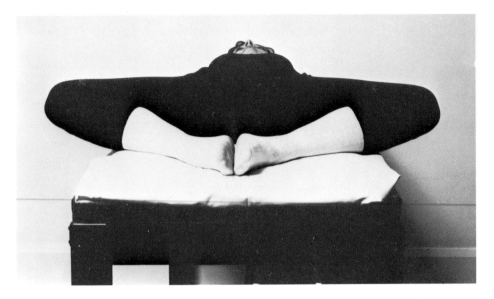

62. Good hip turn out.

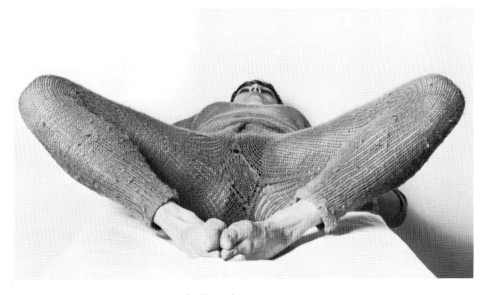

63. Poor hip turn out.

Exercise 1—Hip Rotation:

It is important for a dancer to develop an awareness of the rotary movement possible in the hip joint, and to localise and strengthen the muscles which control this movement. In this way rotatory movement in the hip joint can be isolated from the tipping movement of the pelvis. Stand at the barre and lift one leg forward to 45° with a straight knee, keep the pelvis quite steady, and rotate the whole leg in and out four times, emphasising the out turn. Take the leg into second position and then behind and repeat in these positions. Make sure the pelvis is kept quite steady and repeat with the other leg (Figs. 64, 65).

Exercise 2

This exercise is to help involve the muscles on the inner side of the thighs which are very valuable both in turning out the thigh and in lifting the outwardly rotated leg forwards. In some dancers they remain flabby and unused.

(a) Stand in second position (Fig. 66) and *plié*.
(b) Stick the bottom out.
(c) Stick the bottom in and straighten the knees at the same time push the floor down with the heels. As the knees and thighs come together, the muscles on the inside of the thighs should be felt contracting. Keep repeating the exercise until this is felt (Fig. 67).

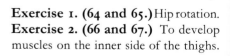

Exercise 1. (64 and 65.) Hip rotation.
Exercise 2. (66 and 67.) To develop muscles on the inner side of the thighs.

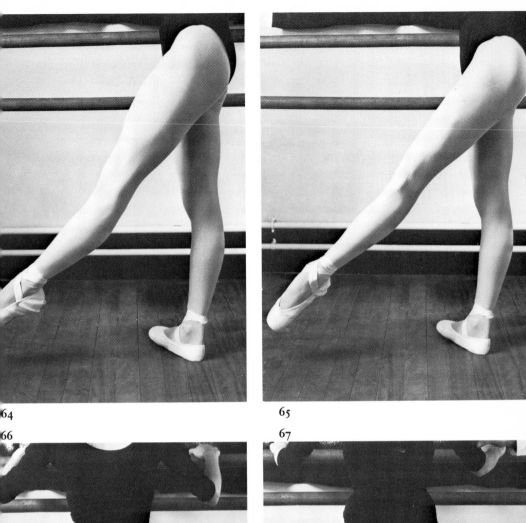

64

65

66

67

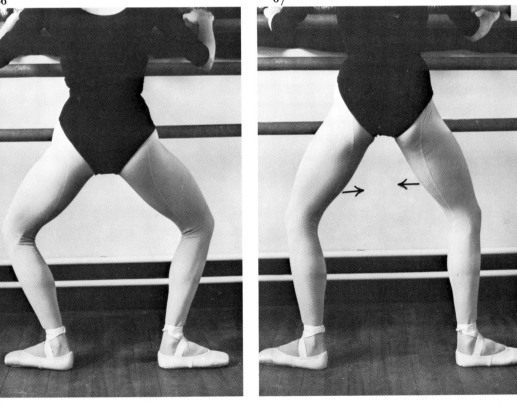

Exercise 3

One important factor that should be known and understood by dancers is that there are two sets of muscles in the sole of the foot responsible for moving the toes:

1. One set come from deep in the calf. They curl the toes under;
2. The other set start within the foot. They pull the knuckles up and straighten the toes.

This exercise is for the short muscles in the sole of the foot. When well developed, these muscles should grip the floor in ballet positions and stop the foot rolling in. With the foot flat on the floor try to pull up the knuckle bones of the toes without curling the toes under—if you curl the toes you are using the wrong muscles (Figs. 68, 69).

If a dancer finds this exercise very difficult the best thing is to have a course of faradic foot baths. These muscles should be used whenever the foot is pointed, i.e. when doing a *tendu*, the ankle joint is first pointed and then the toes are taken over straight with the knuckles coming up (Figs. 70, 71).

Once a dancer is really aware of these valuable muscles in the sole of the foot, the tendons round the ankle joint can be relaxed during a *demi plié* or *fondu,* thus allowing a deeper movement in the ankle joint.

A common problem for dancers is inflammation of the tendons below the inside bone of the ankle joint. This is caused by incorrect use of the long toe muscles from deep in the calf curling the toes to grip the floor at the same time as being stretched in a *fondu.*

Big-Toe Joint

Ideally the big toe should not be much longer than the second toe. The most important thing to notice is how far it bends up towards the ankle joint. Upon this depends how high a dancer will be able to rise on the half point. (See diagram E.)

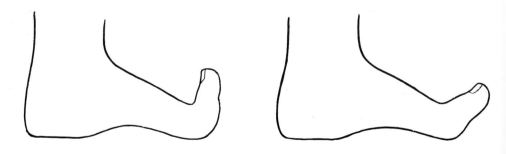

E.
Big toes showing variation in movement.

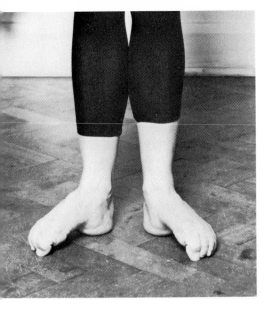

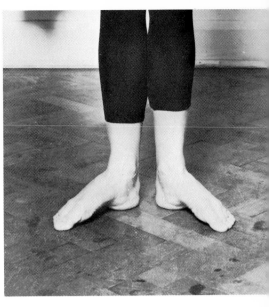

68. Long toe muscles which curl the toes under.

69. Short toe muscles which pull up the knuckles and straighten the toes.

Exercise 3

70 and **71.** A *tendu* using small muscles of the feet.

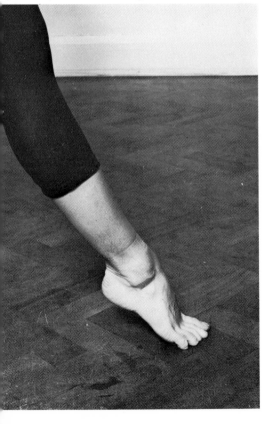

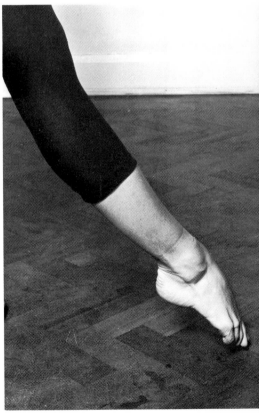

Correct Rise to the Half Point

At first when practising this the dancer's heels should be together and the toes about 90° apart.

There is no better strengthening exercise than slow controlled rises to the half point, BUT there should be no wobbling and the line of weight should go from the centre of the ankle joint to the big toe. This does not mean that the inside arch should be allowed to roll in. On the contrary, it should be kept well up and this is done by keeping the heel forward. Nor should the weight be taken on the outer toes, which are not constructed for weight-bearing (Figs. 72, 73, 74).

One trouble with stiff big-toe joints is that, in an effort to get higher on the half point, the weight is often transferred to the second and third toe joints. Half point work should always be kept at the level of the stiffer joint.

Note to Teachers—When exhorting dancers to rise higher on the half point, they should also be reminded to keep their weight on the big-toe joint.

In the same way on full point the ankle joints should be held firmly and not allowed to sickle in or out (Figs. 75, 76, 77).

Rise to half point

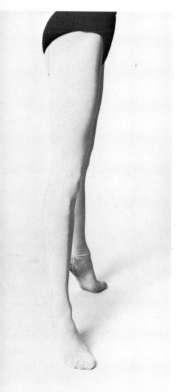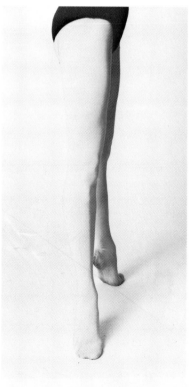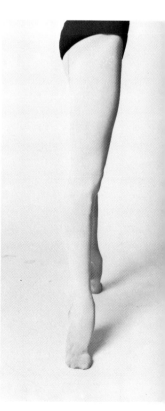

72. Incorrect.   73. Correct.   74. Incorrect.

Rise to full point

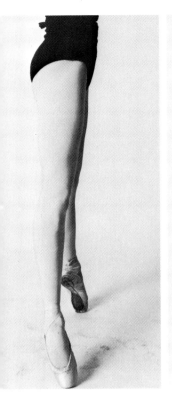 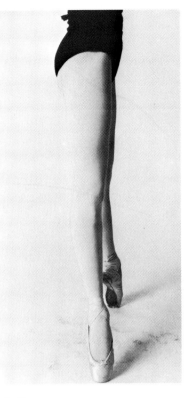 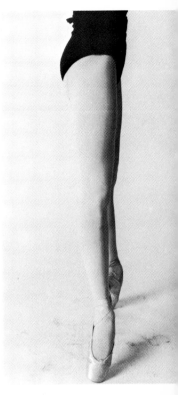

75. Incorrect.   **76.** Correct.   **77.** Incorrect.

Prevention of Stiffness in the Big-Toe Joint

As always, prevention is better than cure. Stiffness is liable to develop in adolescence when the foot is growing rapidly.

Continual stubbing from wearing tight ballet shoes is a predisposing factor (especially if the big toe is longer than the other toes). This problem is more common in boys than in girls, possibly because they wear soft shoes most of the time.

Advice

1. It is a very good idea from time to time to get hold of the big toe and, giving a little traction, move it gently round in circles. Otherwise because of the restricting nature of shoes it tends to get a little stiff, especially in the movement away from the other toes.
2. Don't wear tights and shoes that are too small, and always pull them out at the end to prevent their squashing the toes too much.
3. If pain is felt in this joint don't hesitate to seek advice. Usually rest from

weight-bearing movement, i.e. with a bar on the sole of the shoe, immediately behind but not under the joint is the answer but it is well worth while to let the inflammation settle in this valuable joint.

Bunion

This is the common name for an enlargement on the inner side of the big-toe joint. It is more common in girls than in boys and is made worse by point work. The big toe leans over towards the lesser toes and the bony joint rubs against the shoe, getting red and sore. When it is really inflamed and swollen the bunion is acutely painful, but it does settle down with rest and gives long spells with no trouble at all (Fig. 78).

Ankle Joint

To test the mobility of your ankle joint sit with your feet out in front and your knees straight. Pull your toes up towards the knees and then point them.

The High Arch—The foot with the high arch is beautiful to look at but harder to control. Often with this type of foot the arch is so good that no effort is made to use the small muscles of the foot to take the toes over, and these muscles get neglected (Fig. 79 and Exercise 3, page 42).

One dancer I knew, with a beautiful high arch but a neglected fore-foot, was always working with her weight back on the heels resulting in stiff and aching calf muscles, for which she continually wanted massage. In order to develop the

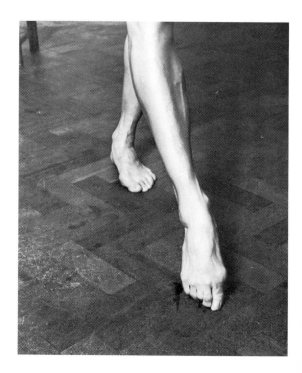

78. Front foot shows bunion. Rear foot shows stretched anterior arch.

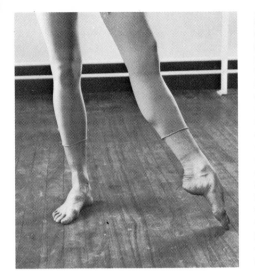

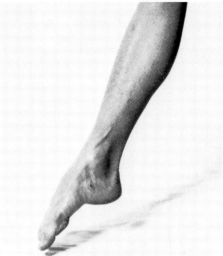

79. A high arch.

80. A low arch.

small muscles in the foot she had to have a month's course of faradic foot baths but since then, with her weight controlled over the fore-foot instead of the heels, the strain has been taken off the calves and massage has virtually become a thing of the past.

It is important with this type of foot to have a firm toe block for point work. I knew another dancer with a similar foot who was in the habit of breaking her shoes so much that, combined with the high arch, her weight was falling too far forward on point. To counteract this she was pulling her weight back and taking the strain below the knee-cap, where she got persistent pain. Luckily the cause was discovered before she had an exploratory operation on her knee-joint!

The Low Arch

If the foot has only a low arch it runs into other problems. A girl can have trouble staying on point without bending the knees a little, which is a very dangerous habit (Fig. 80).

The other problem is pain at the back of the ankle joint caused by compression of one bone on another. This type of foot feels better when it is pulled out and mobilised, and it is also a good idea to do free ankle exercises before starting work, but there is a limit to how much the movement can be increased without damaging the joints.

The Over-Mobile Ankle

Turn the feet in so that the soles face each other, and then out and away from each other (Fig. 81).

Look at them to see if they turn in the same amount. Sometimes after a sprained ankle adhesions will remain round the joint and instep and the foot will not turn in so far, or—and this is more likely with dancers—will turn in further because the ligaments around the outside of the ankle have been damaged and over-stretched. The over-mobile ankle is not a strong structure, and when muscles round the joint get tired it is more likely to become sprained again. It is important to keep the muscles as strong as possible and slow controlled rises to the half point, with no wobbling, are one of the best exercises. It is wise also to keep in reserve an anklet support which can be put on when the dancer feels tired.

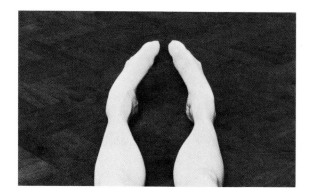

81. Over-mobile ankles (Note the left ankle turns in more than the right).

Straight Leg Raising

Lie flat on your back and lift one leg at a time into the air, keeping the knee quite straight; the distance it goes will depend on the length of the muscles at the back of the thighs (the hamstrings). Long hamstring muscles are a great asset to a dancer (Figs. 82, 83); short hamstring muscles are a great handicap, particularly for a girl. For example, there is a tendency with *grand battements* forwards to allow the lumbar spine to curve backwards in order to get the leg higher in front, and this should be resisted at all costs (Fig. 84). The problem is that it is virtually impossible to stretch the hamstring muscles, and when force is used it is usually the ligaments at the bottom of the back which take the strain. This is weakening for the back and a future cause of trouble in this area. It should be noted here that after an injury to the hamstring muscles it is wise to rest the leg, doing only gentle non-weight-bearing exercises until full range of movement is restored; otherwise, if activity is started too early, a permanent shortening of the hamstring muscle may result.

Leg Length

Very often dancers are told that their back troubles are due to different leg lengths, and this may well be true. Up to half an inch (13mm) difference in length measured

Straight leg raising

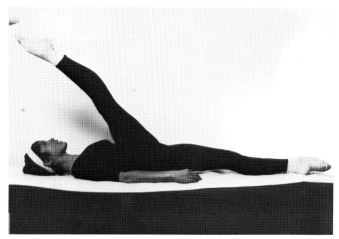

82. Long hamstrings.

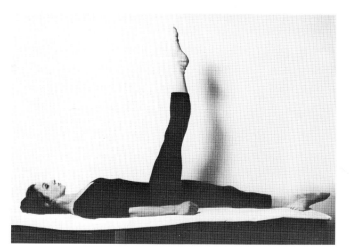

83. Short hamstrings.

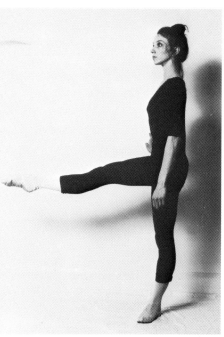

84. *Grand battement* forwards. Note how the short hamstrings cause the lumbar spine to curve backwards.

from the bony prominence on the front of the pelvis to the bone on the inside of the ankle joint is quite normal, and would not be noticed in an ordinary person (Fig. 85), BUT for a dancer even small differences can cause trouble because the longer leg produces uneven pressure on the bottom joint of the spine (lumbo-sacral joint). Aches and pains can result as well as stiffness in the bottom joints of the spine which is restricting for a dancer who is always trying to force each joint to the limit.

There is a temptation for a dancer with stiffness and pain at the bottom of the spine to go for a manipulation; but although temporary relief may be obtained, this is in my experience much more likely to hasten the "wear and tear" symptoms in the lumbo-sacral joint. In general, pains in the spinal joints caused by jarring of the discs are best treated by horizontal rest for the spine, taking the weight off the discs until full movement is restored; this treatment makes recurrence of back trouble less frequent.

Scoliosis

This is a sideways curve in the spine. A curve to the left in the lumbar area invariably means a compensatory curve to the right in the thoracic area. This can be caused by a longer leg, or as in the case of a principal dancer in the Royal Ballet (Figs. 86, 87) by an abnormality in the spine itself. Ballet, with its training in

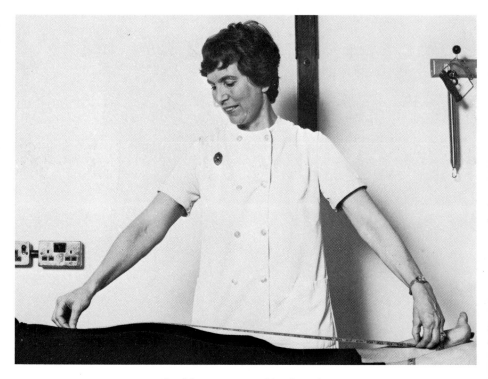

85. Measurement of leg length.

strength and postural sense, is very good treatment for some forms of scoliosis but there will be limitation of movement in the spinal joints. Hanging by the arms is a good way to stretch out and mobilise the spine, as also is swimming.

Scoliosis caused by abnormality in the spine

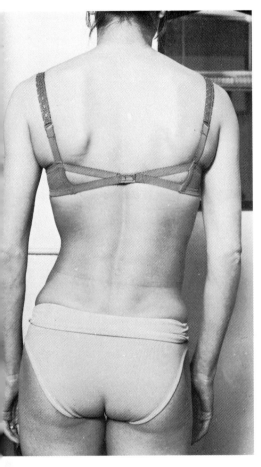

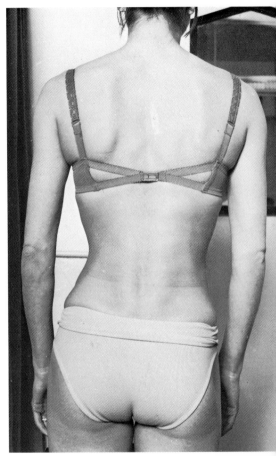

86. Relaxed.

87. Corrected as far as is possible.

Chapter *8*

Hints on Injury Prevention

1. The speed at which you can return to full fitness after a rest period because of vacation or injury will depend on the type of body you have, and your age (see chapter on muscle tone). Although with an older dancer the joints often need a rest, their protection by strong muscles is so important that it is unwise to let the muscles get too unfit.

2. Don't tie ribbons too tight as they can cause irritation of the achilles tendon. If your tendon is sore for any reason, use elastic over the foot to keep on your shoe and temporarily avoid ribbons altogether.

3. Always warm up slowly. It is wise to spend five minutes before a class exercising the feet and ankles to get the blood circulating well to the extremities. *Pliés,* which invariably come at the beginning of a class, are slow controlled exercises, and before doing them it is a good thing to stimulate the circulation to the legs by quick free exercises of the ankles.

4. Don't kneel more than necessary. If this is required by a ballet, wear knee-pads except for the performance. A knee will take so much bruising and no more. In some people the tip of the knee-cap is very sensitive and when it gets bruised it makes all movement of the knee painful.

5. Avoid fatigue if possible, as this is when technique slips and injuries occur. Remember, if you are tired or still growing, to rest the spine lying down whenever possible rather than sitting.

6. Never let the weight of the body rest on the knee-joint in a full *plié,* and if the knee is at all irritable, avoid full *pliés* temporarily.

7. Lifting: Always stand as close to your partner as possible, bending the knees rather than leaning forward from the hips (compare Figs. 20–23 and 88, 89, 90). Lifting is one of the hardest things in ballet and the spine is strongest when it is kept as near to normal upright curves as possible.

8. Ballet exercises are a very hard discipline to return to after an injury, because the basic positions put a big strain on the ligaments of the knees, feet and back. It is wise to work for muscle strength and stamina before pushing the joints to extreme movements. This applies particularly to the turn-out and back movements. Start in a turned-in first position and,

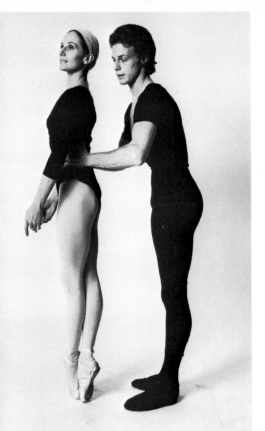

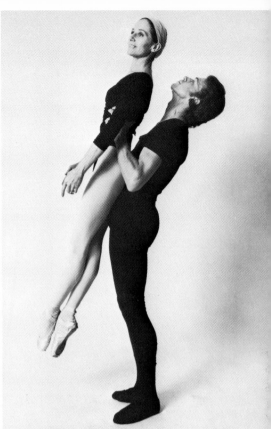

88

89

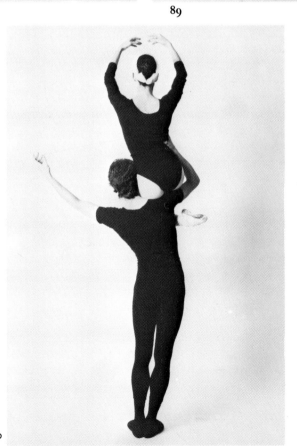

Incorrect lifting

90

when standing on the damaged leg and exercising the good leg, allow the standing foot to face forward; otherwise, exercises, especially in second position, will put a big strain on the damaged weight-bearing leg.

9. Don't ignore stiff calves because stiff muscles are less elastic and more likely to tear. It is all right to work with a raise under the heel, but jumping should be avoided.

10. Try to move each joint in the spine through full movement each day so as to maintain the fullest mobility. Exercises lying down are particularly helpful. When bending backwards, try first to pull the weight up out of the spine so that the discs are compressed as little as possible.

11. Whenever possible keep the head slightly rotated when taking it backwards because this decreases the strain on the base of the neck.

12. When extending the hip in *arabesque* or *grand battement*, keep the leg elongated so that the hamstrings are used for lifting and not just the muscles in the bottom, which otherwise become over-developed.

13. Remember the immediate first aid treatment for most injuries is rest, a firm bandage, and the application of ice to reduce the swelling. Ice cubes wrapped in a polythene bag and a towel are quite an effective method. It is not advisable to continue dancing on the injured part or even to keep it moving because sooner or later the dancer must rest and the more damage there is in the area the more it will swell. After 24–48 hours when there is no danger of increasing the swelling, a good way to stimulate the circulation and so aid recovery is hot and cold contrast baths.

14. It is a good idea to wear soft shoes for barre work so that the small muscles of the foot are felt working against the floor.

15. Dame Margot Fonteyn's advice to young dancers with a good physique is:— If you have an injury give it a chance to recover completely so that you are not left with a weak place which will give recurring trouble. For an older dancer the support strong muscles give to joints is so valuable, it may be necessary to continue limited work with an injury.

Chapter *9*

General Health

The general health of a dancer is of the utmost importance and should be carefully guarded. A dancer's life is very arduous and only with real physical fitness can he (or she) compete in this demanding life.

The biggest factor, which affects so many dancers, is the problem of weight. Many dancers keep their weight below its natural level in order to comply with the demands of ballet. In this case it is important to consult a doctor so that the reduced intake of food gives a balanced diet. Excessive unregulated attempts to reduce weight can have a disastrous effect upon general health and working capacity.

Try to eat a good balanced diet of carbohydrate, fat, and protein, so that the calorie value corresponds to your energy expenditure. There is a tendency, because of weight problems, to eat excessive amounts of protein, which can be detrimental to the body. Carbohydrate intake, on the other hand, should be increased for two days before a big event in order to build up the energy stores in the muscles. (Carbohydrates are contained in potato, cereal, bread, vegetables, fruit, cakes, etc.)

Ideally, food should not be eaten within two hours before a work period; otherwise the digestive organs are vying for the blood which is needed by the muscles. Similarly, food should not be taken within two hours of retiring to bed. This is not an easy rule for dancers to follow because of their long and irregular hours of work.

Natural sources of vitamins are as follows:—

Vitamin
A. Carrots, spinach, cress, liver, kidney, butter, egg yolk.
B. Yeast, wholemeal bread, cereal, wheat germ, eggs.
C. Citrus fruits, green plants.
D. Fish oils, egg yolk, fortified margarine.
E. Fresh vegetables and oils, milk, wheatgerm.

A sufficiency of mineral salts in the diet is also important. Good natural resources are as follows:—

Phosphates   Meat, fish, milk, cheese, carrots, onions, oatmeal, wheat, peas, beans.

Iron	Liver, strawberries, spinach, eggs, kidneys, raisins, wholemeal bread.
Calcium	Milk, cheese, white bread.
Magnesium	Cheese, oatmeal, beans, peas.
Sodium and Potassium chloride	General diet.

Fluid Intake

Water intake should be on average $3\frac{1}{2}$–$4\frac{1}{2}$ pints per day (including the water in food). This water is generally excreted in the form of urine. An athlete can lose profuse quantities in sweating, especially in a hot climate, and he may need two pints a day extra fluid to allow for this. Water is often more acceptable if it is slightly acidified with lemon juice. Extra salt may be needed in the diet or in the form of salt tablets, as lack of salt can cause muscle cramps, but in fact salt depletion is rare compared with dehydration and too much salt will just make the dancer unnecessarily thirsty.

Smoking

Unfortunately smoking seems to be a hazard of a dancer's life, because of the atmosphere of tension, and the boredom of rehearsals, but it is a damaging habit and should be resisted from the beginning. Nicotine, besides introducing poison into the system, irritates the air tubes going to the lungs causing them to thicken and become less elastic. This means that with exertion, oxygen intake is restricted, making the dancer more breathless than he (or she) would otherwise be.

Some of the information in this chapter was derived from an article by Mr M. Down in the British Journal of Sports Medicine.

Chapter *10*

Non-Weight-Bearing Exercises

There are often times when a dancer is unable to do class or even barre work because of an injury, and at these times non-weight-bearing exercises can be a great help in maintaining some degree of fitness. Also it is a good thing to mobilise joints and strengthen muscles without the weight of the body.

The eight exercises described below are just a few of many. Not all of them will necessarily be suitable in each case; so a dancer should select those that cause no pain to the injured area.

Each exercise should be repeated six times to begin with, increasing to twelve times.

Exercise 1. For the upper back (Fig. 91).

The dancer lies on her tummy with pillows under her hips, and lifts up her head and shoulders arching the upper back and turning her arms out.

91

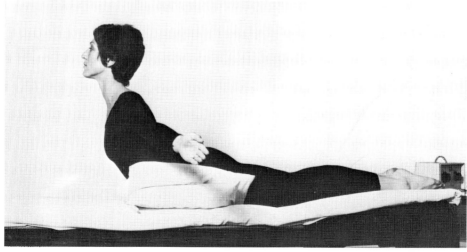

Exercise 2. For the lower back and hips (Figs. 92, 93)

The dancer lies as in exercise 1 and lifts one leg backwards and then the other, keeping the knee straight. Then both legs are lifted together. If this causes pain in the lower back don't lift the legs so high.

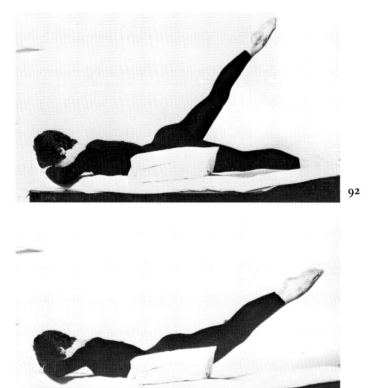

92

93

Exercise 3. For the hips (Fig. 94).

The dancer lies on her side with the underneath leg bent. She lifts the upper leg sideways and then lowers it keeping the knee straight.

This exercise can be varied by taking the upper leg round in circles.

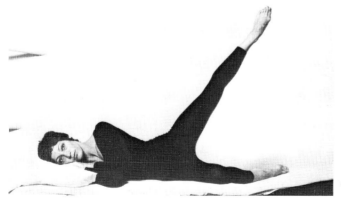

94

Exercise 4. For the abdominal muscles (Figs. 95, 96, 97).

The dancer lies on her back with her knees bent and her arms stretched above her head. Reaching forward with her arms she slowly sits up straight and then places her hands behind her neck. Her back should be straight and her elbows back. She then reaches her arms forwards and slowly lowers her back joint by joint until she is lying flat again with her arms above her head.

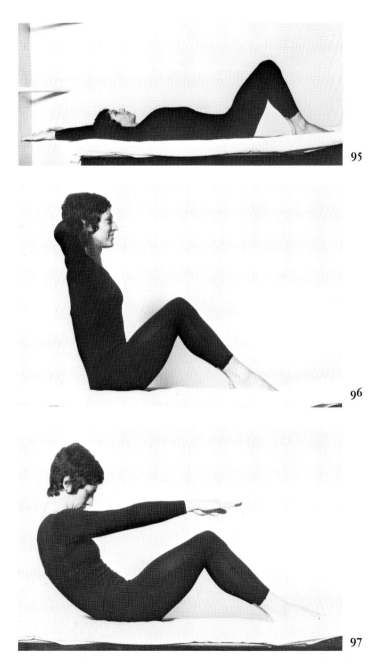

95

96

97

Exercise 5. For the abdominal muscles and hips (Figs. 98, 99).

The dancer lies flat and then lifts both legs together, keeping the knees straight, until they are vertical. The legs are then dropped sideways, brought together again and lowered onto the bed.

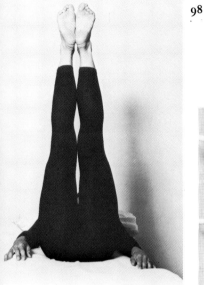

98

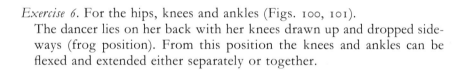

99

Exercise 6. For the hips, knees and ankles (Figs. 100, 101).

The dancer lies on her back with her knees drawn up and dropped sideways (frog position). From this position the knees and ankles can be flexed and extended either separately or together.

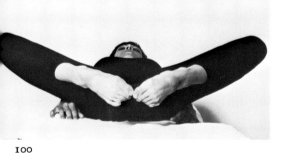

100

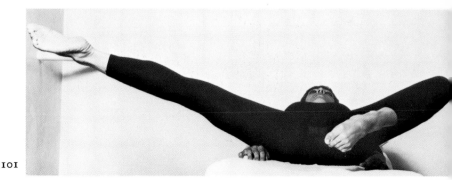

101

Exercise 7. For the back and thighs (Figs. 102, 103).

The dancer kneels with her head on the bed and her bottom separated from her heels by a pillow. She then kneels up straight arching the upper back and turning her arms out above her head. She then returns to a curled up position with her arms behind her back.

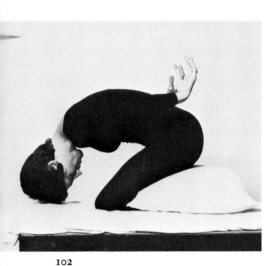

102

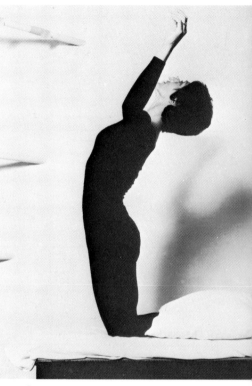

103

Exercise 8. For the back and hips (especially good for the "turn-out" muscles in the hips) (Figs. 104, 105, 106).

The dancer kneels on all fours; that is with the knees and arms on the bed, and the spine horizontal.

(1)   She bends one knee to touch her head.
(2)   She lifts up her head and takes her hip sideways keeping the knee bent.
(3)   She stretches the leg up backwards straightening the knee.
(4)   She returns to position (2).
(5)   Then to position (1).
(6)   Then to the starting position.
      Repeat with the other leg.

Breathing exercises as described on pages 31 and 32 are always advisable; also exercises for the small muscles of the feet as described on page 42.

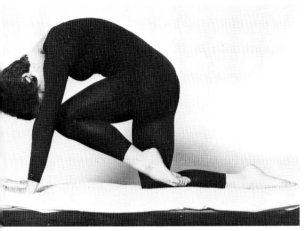

104

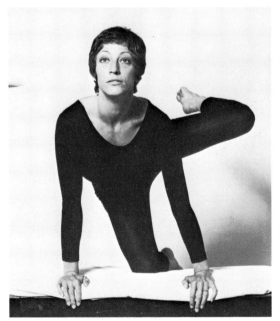

105

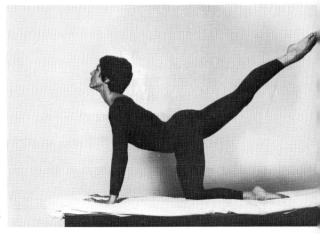

106

Chapter *II*

Treatment

The Royal Ballet Company consists of seventy female and fifty-five male dancers. It is divided into a main company, and a smaller touring company which spends most of its time in the provinces or abroad giving 8 performances a week. The main company, which is based in London, gives an average of 3–4 performances a week but the dancers also spend up to six hours a day training or rehearsing. The daily class usually lasts one and a half hours; half an hour of this is spent doing exercises holding onto a barre, and the next hour is spent in the centre of the studio doing slow controlled and quicker jumping exercises. Barre work is often thought of as a gentle form of rehabilitation but in fact these exercises take the body through all the extreme range of movement of classical ballet and this is not always the best thing after an injury (Figs. 107, 108, 109).

The physiotherapy treatment room was set up at the Royal Ballet School, where class and rehearsals take place, in 1959. It is a large room in which dancers are able to get advice and on-the-spot treatment. There are great advantages in having a room on the premises as it means that dancers can come for treatment between or during rehearsals when they are free. There is strong pressure on dancers not to miss rehearsals even on medical grounds, partly from the management and partly from the dancers themselves who are afraid of losing a coveted role.

It is hard to imagine without working within a ballet company the amount of work which goes into producing the grace and mastery of movement which is the basis of a ballet performance. The pressure on both staff and dancers is tremendous. If a dancer is suddenly unable to perform, a whole ballet may have to be re-rehearsed at the last moment.

Another advantage of having a treatment room adjoining the studio is that strains will often occur in class work where technique is being pushed to the limit. Injuries tend to occur more often during a rehearsal than in a performance, because of the endless repetition in a struggle for perfection. Learning a new role is particularly hazardous because the complicated co-ordination has not become automatic (Figs. 110, 111, 112, 113, 114).

Thus ballet dancers are by the very nature of their work exposed to many injuries or strains. Most people whose livelihood depends on physical performance can, with first aid and a little determination, carry on in spite of an injury. But a dancer needs a full range of movement in every joint, and anything which interferes with this impairs his ability to perform. Also, dancing with an injury almost invariably produces a second injury or strain. Thus the consequences of injury for dancers are quite serious. When these factors are considered in relation to a group of people who have both a heightened awareness of their bodies and state of physical fitness and a tendency towards "artistic temperament", it will be readily understood that injuries, real or less real, frequently create a sense of urgency, tension and fear.

The correlation between, on the one hand variation in physique and errors in technique, and on the other the commonly recurring strains and injuries in ballet dancers makes a fascinating study. With experience it is quite possible by examining a dancer's physique to predict not only those who will be prone to injuries, but also the injuries or strains from which they are most likely to suffer.

Barre work

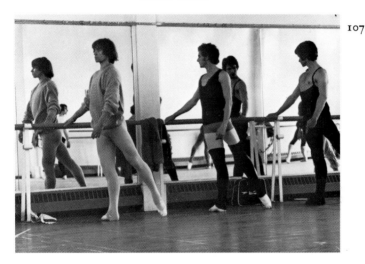

107

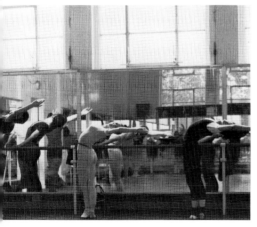

108

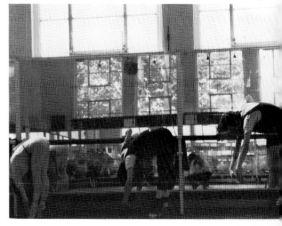

109

Class work

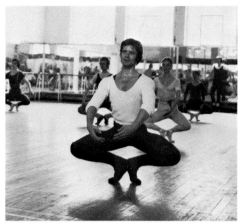

110

111

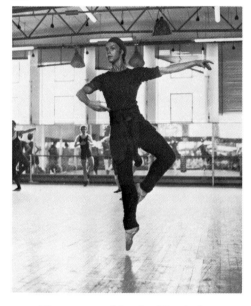

112

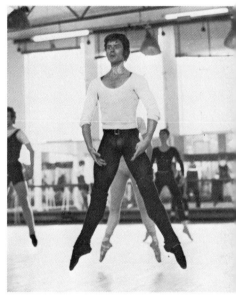

Those treated in the Physiotherapy room fall largely into three groups:

1. Dancers who require minor treatment and reassurance, and who can continue dancing.
2. Dancers who in addition to treatment require their work to be restricted, and possibly even a short period of complete rest.
3. Dancers with more serious injuries. These are sent to the consultant orthopaedic surgeon, who also pays a weekly visit to check and advise on minor ailments.

Naturally, as with all athletes, the most important thing is an accurate assessment of the injury or strain. It is a great advantage to know the personality of the dancer and something of the demands to be made on him or her. Often a dancer in the *corps de ballet* can carry on when a principal dancer will have to rest. Because of the psychological distress caused by any limitation in activities, if any injury or strain does warrant cancellation of rehearsals or performances, a dancer should be given very clear instructions as to what he should and should not do in order to gain the quickest recovery. It is important to understand that most dancers are totally immersed in the art of dancing and if this is interfered with, a step-by-step detailed recovery programme must be worked out with the therapist. As a general rule, when a dancer re-starts after an injury he should allow a period at least as long as his absence before he can count himself as fit. It is essential that management should also be involved in these decisions and that they too are aware of what is best for the dancer.

In the remainder of this chapter the commonly recurring strains and injuries directly related to ballet dancing will be described and discussed. In each case treatment which has proved most beneficial to dancers of the Royal Ballet Company over the past 14 years will be suggested. It is always important to check if there is anything in the physique or technique which has contributed towards the injury or strain. Nine times out of ten this will be the case, so that besides treating the present condition advice should be given on preventing recurrence.

The equipment in the physiotherapy room is as follows: short wave diathermy, ultrasound, faradic machine, heat tunnel, heat lamp, massage machines, traction apparatus, hydrocolator for heating hot packs, chemical ice packs, electric blanket, weights, overhead slings, a barre, improved equipment for giving resistance to invertor and evertor muscles of the foot (Fig. 117), 3 plinths, and hot and cold water.

Medical and Surgical Supplies include:
1. Orthopaedic felt—various thicknesses.
2. Elastoplast strapping (Poroplast has the advantage of being skin coloured).
3. Elastoplast with dressings.
4. Crepe bandages.
5. Sponge rubber for making heel pads.
6. Sponge rubber collars—(sponge rubber 1 in. thick covered by stockinette or gauze).
7. Collection of adjustable corsets.
8. Sticks and crutches.
9. Surgical spirit and powder.
10. TCP or antiseptic lotion.
11. Calgene massage cream (Calmic Ltd).
12. Witch hazel.
13. Brusol (Calmic Ltd) for bruises.
14. Methocarbamol (Robaxin) for muscle spasm.
15. Soluble codeine.
16. Sleeping pills (used very stringently).

The following *Home Treatments* are frequently advised:
1. Application of ice cubes wrapped in a polythene bag and towel and applied to the injured part for 20 minutes every 2–3 hours. This is very effective in preventing and reducing swelling.
2. Contrast baths. These are a very effective way of stimulating the circulation before exercises for a more chronic injury, particularly in the lower leg where the foot can be immersed in a basin of hot water for 2 minutes and held under the cold tap for $\frac{1}{2}$ minute and the process repeated several times.

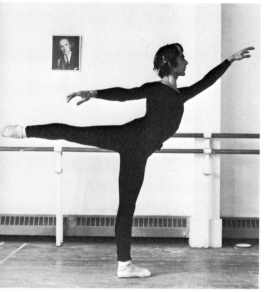
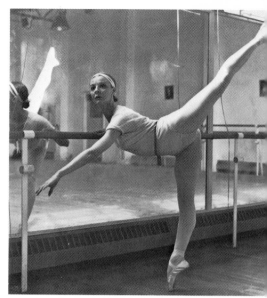

113. Donald Macleary in first *arabesque*   **114.** Antoinette Sibley in second *arabesque*.

Dancer's Chart

Opposite is the chart I have devised whereby I can examine and keep a record of the physical details of each dancer. Joint movement is measured and compared with the other side of the body. Potential problems can be detected, and advice given on posture, mobilising and strengthening. In this way injury and strain can often be avoided.

COMMON STRAINS AND INJURIES AMONGST DANCERS

FEET

Hallux Valgus:

This is disabling because it causes extra wear and tear on the medial side of the big-toe joint and is associated with stretching of the anterior arch (Fig. 78) p. 46.

Short wave diathermy, passive gentle mobilisation, and faradic foot baths are given. Sometimes, a small metatarsal pad to lift the stretched anterior arch will help to draw together the metatarsal heads and so take pressure off the big-toe joint. This can be combined with some strapping round the forefoot if the dancer can tolerate it.

Bunion:

If this is acutely inflamed the important thing is to keep pressure off it. This can sometimes be done with felt padding but it usually means complete rest from dancing and wearing a large low-heeled shoe. Surprisingly, even acutely inflamed bunions settle down and give long periods without trouble.

NAME			AGE 20	HEIGHT 5' 1½"	WEIGHT 7st 2lb
FEET	RIGHT	LEFT	REMARKS		
BIG TOE FLEX. 90°	90°	−10°	Left foot little longer		
BUNION	−	Slight			
TRANSVERSE ARCH	3rd ↓	3rd ↓	Mobile arch		
TARSAL-METATARSAL	−	+5°			
INVERSION	√	√	Normal		
EVERSION	√	√			
DORSIFLEXION 90°	+10°	+10°			
PLANTARFLEX 180°	+5°	180°			
S.L.R. 90°	+25°	+25°			
SHAPE LEG	Straight				
MED. ROT. PATELLA FEET VERTICAL	−	−			
LEG LENGTH	31¼"	31¼"			
HIPS					
FLEXION	√	√			
INTERNAL ROT.	20°	15°			
EXT. ROT. FROG POS.	55°	55°			
ABDUCTION	60°	60°			
EXTENSION PR. LY.	55°	65°			
SHOULDERS	√	√			
BACK			Tends to stand with lumbar kyphosis		
SIDE FLEX.	√	√			
ROTATION	√	√			
FLEXION	Little stiff in thoracic area				
EXTENSION	√	√			
LENGTH OF BODY TOP OF HEAD TO PUBIC SYMPHYSIS	30½ inches				
LENGTH OF LEGS PUBIC SYMPHYSIS TO GROUND	31 inches				

This dancer needs a little posture correction and exercises for her left intrinsic foot muscles. Otherwise very good.

Dropped metatarsal heads:

This is often associated with the above conditions and is best treated by faradism and a pad. When giving faradism to the feet it is a good idea to put one electrode under the heel and the other under the four outer toes but *not* under the big toe, as this will often cause cramping of the stronger muscles under the medial arch. I have also found that covering the electrodes with damp lint is preferable to a foot bath (Fig. 115).

Always check the mobility of the big-toe joint and the correct rise to half point. Almost invariably pain under the anterior arch is associated with an incorrect rise, either because of stiffness or pain in the big-toe joint or weakness of the ankle muscles.

Real stability is only acquired when the line of weight is taken from the centre of the ankle joint to the big toe. When rising to half point make sure the heel is kept forward as this stops the medial arch rolling in.

Stress fracture of metatarsal:

The usual place for this to take place is the neck of the bone just proximal to the head. Sudden pain particularly with jumping, and local tenderness should arouse suspicion. On the other hand tenderness on the metatarsal head is usually caused

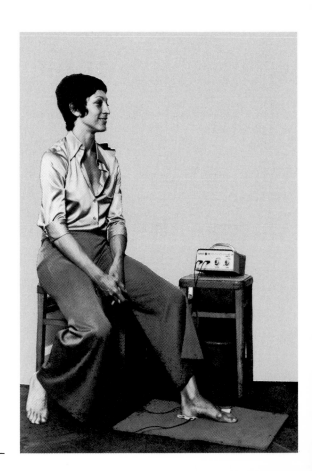

115. Faradism for the small muscles of the feet.

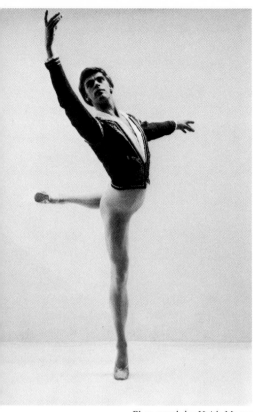

116. Christopher Gable in *attitude croisé* on half point following a Keller's operation.

Photograph by Keith Money

by bruising. Early X-rays will often not show a crack but if a fracture is suspected it is worth taking one because if it does show, confirmation can be given that no jumping will be possible for three weeks.

Hallux Rigidus:

This form of arthritis in the 1st metatarsal-phalangeal joint of the big toe usually starts in adolescence and, as discussed on page 45, prevention would be easier than cure. It seems to be commoner in boys than girls, possibly because male dancers wear soft and tightly fitting shoes most of the time; this must lead to continual mild trauma of the big toe.

It is a great disability for a dancer as it limits the height to which he can rise correctly on half point. If there is a variation in stiffness of the big-toe joints, always check that half point is kept to the height allowed by the stiffest joint. Heat, ultrasound, frictions, and passive mobilisation may help the chronic joint but any injury causing an acute flare-up should be treated with great respect and rested until the inflammation has subsided. I have known two male dancers both with severe bilateral hallux rigidus who have had Keller's operation, and returned to full work with much improved technique after six months. One of them, at the age of 19 years, had enlarged and inflamed big toe joints with only $2°-3°$ painful movement in each. They had been like that for several years but afraid he would be told to give up he had persevered, taking the weight on the 2nd and 3rd metatarsal heads. Six to twelve months after the operation the biggest change he noticed was the increase in strength of his whole body as weight was transmitted correctly to the big-toe joints (Fig. 116).

Strained insertion of peroneus brevis:

Tenderness over the base of the fifth metatarsal and pain with eversion is a very disabling injury for a dancer because the muscle is used so much for rising and balancing. It means that all forms of ballet work will irritate it and delay recovery.

Fracture of the base of the 5th metatarsal:

Even with a crack without displacement it is better to keep weight off the foot for six weeks; otherwise it has been found that the pull of the tendons on the fracture site, even with walking, seems to delay bony healing. This also precludes non-weight-bearing exercises for the foot, which means that when the fracture is really firm recovery of muscle strength and co-ordination will take another four to six weeks. With a more severe fracture complete immobilisation in plaster of Paris is very important until bony union is evident.

Strain at Tarso-metatarsal joint:

The dorsal ligaments of the tarso-metatarsal joints are quite often stretched in point work so that some plantar-flexion takes place at these joints. This can happen

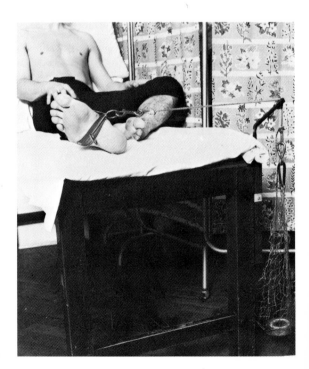

117. Resisted eversion exercises.

in a foot with loose ligaments, or in a firmer foot with a stiff ankle, which transfers strain to this area.

Ultrasound and frictions should help and when the acute symptoms have subsided manipulations will prevent adhesions. Elastoplast strapping round the forefoot is often helpful.

INVERSION SPRAIN OF THE ANKLE JOINT

1. Sprain of the lateral ligament of the ankle joint:

The majority of lateral ligament sprains involve no fracture. Usually there is tenderness over the lower end of the fibula, swelling round the anterior lateral ligament, and pain here if the foot is inverted. Immediate application of ice, a firm bandage and elevation of the foot is the best early treatment. This should be continued for 24–48 hours according to the severity of the injury. It is quite hard to persuade a dancer to keep the foot off the ground—that is to use crutches for unavoidable walking, but this greatly shortens the recovery time. Non-weight-bearing exercises should be done in elevation when the initial acuteness has subsided, but crutches should be used until swelling has gone out of the ankle joint. Otherwise, early weight-bearing activity tends to leave not only a chronic lump of thickening round the lateral malleolus, but also persistent tenderness of the lower end of the fibula, both of which will restrict full range of movement in the ankle and delay full recovery.

After a few days the patient will almost invariably complain of pain below the medial malleolus, presumably where the structures were jarred during the sprain. Ultrasound and massage to both sides of the joint below the malleoli will help to reduce swelling and bruising, but ultrasound has not been found helpful over the lower end of the fibula where the periosteum is sore. After 24–48 hours heat may be given or a hot bath before non-weight-bearing exercises. Resisted exercises are delayed until all soreness has gone from the periosteum. Faradic foot baths are started fairly soon but the main thing is to keep weight off the joint until all the swelling has gone.

X-ray: This involves a visit to hospital or a private clinic so unless the injury is very severe it is often delayed a few days until the initial symptoms have subsided, because of the importance of immediate elevation of the foot.

2. Sprain of the lateral dorsal ligaments of tarsal bones:

When landing from a jump with the foot pointed, the strain is often taken on the lateral dorsal ligaments of the tarsal bones rather than the lateral ligaments of the ankle joint. The prognosis of recovery is quicker with this injury, and it is treated in the same way except that crutches are less important if there is no swelling in the ankle joint.

3. Severe sprain of the ankle:

This is more common in men landing from a big jump. Besides partial rupture of the lateral ligament, there can also be some tearing of the inferior tibia-fibular ligament with additional swelling over the front of the ankle. This is a more serious injury and probably will mean six weeks off weight-bearing and possibly a spell in plaster. A complete rupture of the lateral ligament possibly requiring re-constructive surgery has not been seen in this department.

Strained insertion of tibialis posterior or tibialis anterior:

Ultrasound and finger massage usually help and possibly some Elastoplast support. Always check for possible errors in technique: (i) that the medial arch is not being allowed to roll in when the dancer rises to half point; (ii) that when standing in first position the medial arch is held by the intrinsic muscles gripping the floor and NOT by overworking the tibialis anterior or posterior tendons which will tend to lift the big-toe joint off the ground. Both these faults will predispose towards the above injury. If necessary, faradism for the intrinsic foot muscles should be recommended.

Tenosynovitis of the flexor hallucis longus and flexor digitorum longus tendons:

Pain and swelling below and behind the medial malleolus is quite common. As discussed on page 42 this usually comes from overwork of the long flexors in gripping the floor. There may be no pain on resisted toe flexion but the last few degrees of pointing the feet give pain. On freely flexing and extending the toes a fine crepitus may be felt below and behind the medial malleolus. This means an acute inflammation and is treated with mild ultrasound and rest. On the other hand a loud click denotes a chronic condition temporarily made worse. (Sometimes even a loud clicking will give no trouble at all.) Both conditions should be given faradism for the small foot muscles if necessary.

Tenosynovitis or tendinitis of the tibialis posterior:

This tendon bears a heavy load with continual rising, jumping and balancing. Extra strain is added if the foot rolls in at all because of fatigue or because the foot has turned out beyond the knee. If there is any bowing in the lower leg the line of weight will not fall centrally through the ankle joint and will throw more strain on the structures supporting the inside arch. This is a problem to be lived with but it is important to keep the intrinsic muscles strong and limit turn-out for a time.

Usually when the tendon sheath is inflamed and thickened there is *no* pain with active contraction of the tendon.

Ankle Joint:

(i) Pain over the antero-lateral joint line:
With no history of sprain the cause is almost certainly bruising of the synovium or capsule. This comes from using the ankle hinge-joint unevenly during a *plié* or *fondu*, because the feet are turned out beyond the knees, thus overcompressing the antero-lateral part of the joint. Ultrasound and mobilisation with traction will help but technique must be watched (Fig. 118).

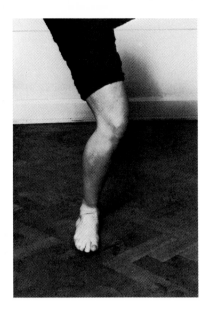

118. Note the mal-alignment between the knee and the ankle.

(ii) Arthritic changes along anterior joint line:

This can occur in an older dancer or one who has been forcing dorsiflexion beyond the natural limit. It is caused by continual trauma between the lower anterior border of the tibia and the upper surface of the talus. Ultrasound and a spell off jumping and deep *fondus* is advised. Sometimes a hydrocortisone injection will give relief but this may well increase joint deterioration in the long run and is not recommended. Pain with a *fondu* presents a problem because very soon the dancer starts tensing the calf muscles when landing from a jump.

Extensor retinaculum:

Pain on the lower end of the tibia just anterior to the medial malleolus is not uncommon amongst male dancers. There is a tenderness on the bone and pain with a *fondu* (Diagram F). This seems to be periostitis caused by pulling of the extensor

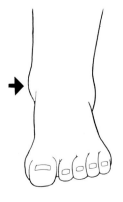

F.
Diagram showing medial attachment of anterior retinaculum.

retinaculum when it is stretched forward during a *fondu* and jumping. It is difficult to help this except by rest and it will tend to recur. A complication of working with this injury is strain in the achilles tendon as the dancer resists putting his heels down.

Dancer's Heel:

This is an expression we have coined to describe pain in the posterior part of the talo-calcaneal joint, which is quite a common problem with dancers. It is more common in girls and seems to be associated with much point work on hard floors. Pain is produced by active and passive full plantar-flexion unless traction is given to the calcaneum. The prone position with the knee bent to 90° is a good one in which to hold the calcaneum away from the talus. In this way full plantar-flexion can be quite painless (Fig. 119). A good way to test the limitation of plantar-flexion is to lay a dancer face down with the ankles supported over a pillow and just push the heels up. If movement is limited it will show clearly in this position. It is as if the articular cartilage has become bruised and swollen, and relief is given if the joints are held apart. When plantar-flexion is limited, it is difficult for the dancer to stand on point without bending the knees. Ultrasound treatment may help but usually a dancer needs to spend several weeks on a flat foot with no rises, or rises only as far as to cause no pain.

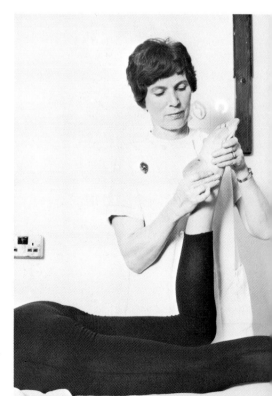

119. Mobilisation of the talocalcaneal joint.

Os trigonum:

Persistent pain behind the ankle joint is an indication for X-ray as it is not uncommon to find a small bone restricting full plantar-flexion and causing inflammation. This can be removed surgically and full recovery takes about three months. Results have usually been quicker when the incision is on the medial rather than the lateral side of the ankle. This seems to be because ballet positions make it easier to stretch scar tissue on the medial side of the foot.

Bursae:

Deep to the achilles tendon a bursa can become swollen and is usually helped by ultrasound or by a hydrocortisone injection. Superficially a bursa over the achilles insertion can become inflamed from pressure. This will usually settle when external pressure is removed, but a very bad one can be removed surgically.

THE LOWER LEG:

Stress fracture of the tibia:

This is a very important injury to check for. The dancer, usually male, complains

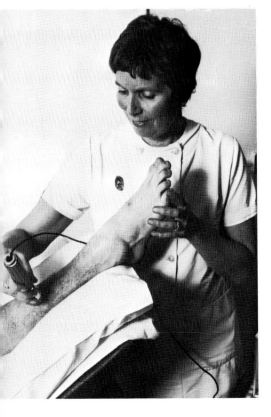

120. Ultrasound treatment given in elevation.

of pain and aching in the shin with jumping and there is local tenderness on the middle of the shin. This tenderness is confined to the bone. Diagnosis should be made from these clinical symptoms, as nothing may show on an X-ray for several months. If treated early there may be no need to take the dancer off weight-bearing, but it is very important to stop ALL forms of ballet, even barre exercises, for three months. In our experience several stress fractures have occurred in dancers within a few weeks of returning to work after a month's holiday. My view is that jumping at the beginning of the season with the feet turned out, but without proper control of the hips, causes a rotation stress on the tibia which is a contributing factor.

Tibialis Anterior:

If some muscle fibres are torn there will be local tenderness lateral to the shin bone and pain with inversion, but this should settle fairly quickly with ultrasound and rest. Acute stiffness or hypertrophy of these muscles is very painful owing to the swelling in a small compartment. Mild ultrasound in elevation seems to be the most helpful treatment (Fig. 120).

The medial border of the tibia:

Tenderness along the lower half of the medial border of the tibia is not uncommon. The symptoms are pain with jumping, and aching afterwards. It seems to be caused by a periostitis where the calf muscle fascia has pulled on its attachment to the medial border of the tibia. It is more likely to occur if the dancer has done an extra amount of jumping and turned the feet out too far. No physiotherapy treatment really helps but barre work should be done "turned in", avoiding *fondus* and, of course, jumping, till the tenderness settles.

Fibula:

Surprisingly, fractures of this bone are rare. It is quite common for a dancer to have pain with jumping and local tenderness on the lateral border of the fibula about 2 inches (5 cm) above the malleolus, but in my experience with two exceptions X-ray has never shown a fracture. A possible cause is irritation of the periosteum by the shoe-ribbons. It usually settles with a week's rest from jumping, and it is a good idea to protect the fibula with padding under ribbons.

Calf muscles:

As always, prevention of trouble is better than cure, and acutely stiff calf muscles should be given immediate treatment. Massage is always a treatment in demand but sometimes the muscles are too tender to tolerate this, and ultrasound has been found to be very effective. Often ten minutes of ultrasound to one calf muscle (strength varying with the acuteness of the stiffness) can reduce a really tense muscle to a soft flaccid one. The most helpful advice is to wear shoes with a good heel and, if possible, stop jumping; in any case a pad of sponge rubber under the heel is a help. A gentle method of stretching the calf muscles is shown in Fig. 121.

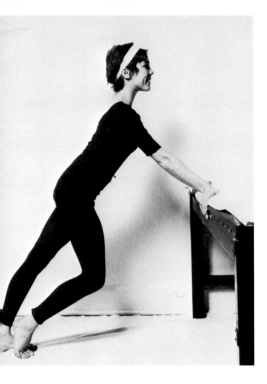

121. Gentle stretch for the calves and achilles tendon.

Tear in the belly of the muscle :

The immediate treatment is an ice pack, rest, and wearing a high heel. Mild ultra-sound can be started straight away or in a day or two, depending on the severity of the injury. No heat or massage should be given because of the danger of increasing bleeding at the site. Once a haematoma has formed ultrasound seems to be the most effective treatment in helping it to disperse, together with non-weight-bearing exercises.

Strained musculo-tendinous junction :

This, being the weakest part of the calf, is by far the commonest site of strain; it is not so acute as a tear in the vascular muscle fibres but it is disabling because pain causes the whole calf to seize up. Fairly strong ultrasound given locally to the musculo-tendinous junction has been found most helpful.

The range of movement of the calf muscles should be checked, taking the foot into dorsiflexion with the knee bent and straight. It is a good idea to resist plantar-flexion in both these positions before taking the foot into dorsiflexion as the muscles relax. The result of this test gives a good idea of the severity of the injury and it also keeps the maximum passive stretch in the muscle. Fig. 121 shows gentle stretch to achilles tendon and calf.

Ruptured achilles tendon :

We have had only two cases in fourteen years, both in dancers aged over 30 years who have done a great deal of jumping. Both tendons were sutured, and the dancers have returned to full work, though heavy jumping roles have not been encouraged! Treatment will vary according to the orthopaedic surgeon, but in principle when weight-bearing is allowed after six weeks, it is better to work for strength with weight-bearing exercises with no stretch on the tendon, i.e. rises but no *fondus*; and use non-weight-bearing exercises gently to stretch the tendon; i.e. during a *plié* keep all the weight on the good leg. It will be found that as the tendon gets stronger and thinner it will allow more stretch (Figs. 122, 123).

122 and **123.** *Fondu* following a ruptured left achilles tendon. Note the deeper *fondu* on the right leg.

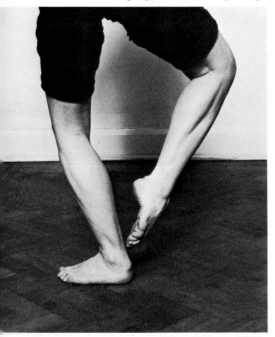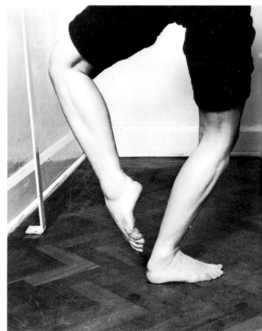

Peritendinitis of the achilles tendon:

This is not as common as one would expect, considering the amount of calf work and the added factor of ballet ribbons, which are usually tied too tightly above the ankle joint, but pain with a fine crepitus must be treated by rest, usually for a week after all symptoms have subsided.

Tendinitis:

Inflammation of the tendon itself tends to occur with overwork, especially if the dancer has tight achilles tendons and is unable to get her heels down in jumping.

There is no creaking but the tendon is very sore to touch. Sometimes a few fibres are torn and there is a little lump of inflammation. Rest is the important treatment with a heeled shoe until the inflammation has settled.

Local injection of hydrocortisone is not recommended, because, although it may reduce the painful inflammatory reaction in the injured area, it may also interfere with natural healing and will render the part liable to severe injury if strain is put on the structure.

Likewise an injection of local anaesthetic may easily mean the conversion of a partial to a complete tear.

KNEE JOINT:

With all knee injuries it is wise to check for wasting of the quadriceps 1 inch (25mm) and 4 inches (100mm) above the upper border of the patella.

Torn Meniscus:

This injury is the dread of every dancer but, surprisingly enough, during the fourteen years I have worked with the Royal Ballet Company of over 100 dancers only three have had a meniscectomy. At least another half dozen, whose symptoms have been ascribed to torn meniscus by several orthopaedic surgeons, have with palliative treatment recovered and continued normal work. It appears that the meniscus can be pulled a little off the tibia causing swelling and limited movement in the joint and sometimes a positive McMurray's click but, given a chance, it can re-attach itself and the knee settles down again.

Because of this I like to treat knees with suspected meniscus injuries with as little movement to the joint as possible to begin with. The knee is rested in a splint, and faradism is given to the quadriceps and possibly short wave diathermy to the knee joint. The splint is kept on until any swelling has gone and there is full extension in the knee joint. Straight leg raising exercises are given and resistance added. For strengthening the quadriceps anti-gravity exercises have been found more satisfactory than weight-lifting because of the strain on the lower end of the patella.

Quadriceps exercises:

(i)   Keep the knees and feet together and bend the knees, lifting the heels at the same time. Straighten the knees and then lower the heels (Fig. 124, 125, 126).

(ii) Step on and off a stool on one leg, then rise on to the toes and firmly pull up the knee (Figs. 127, 128).

Strains of the Medial and Coronary ligaments:

These injuries for dancers have the added disadvantage that all forms of ballet work put a strain on the damaged structures which means that recovery from the work point of view takes longer. Ultrasound and frictions are usually helpful and it is important to keep the quadriceps as strong as possible with non-ballet exercises.

Quadriceps exercises

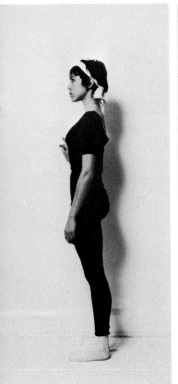

124

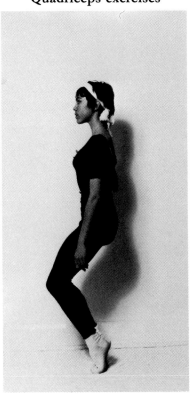

125

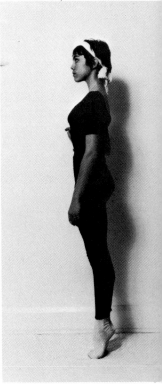

126

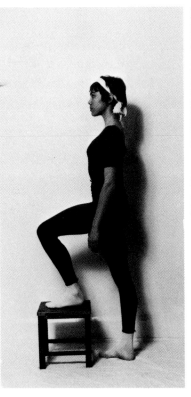

127

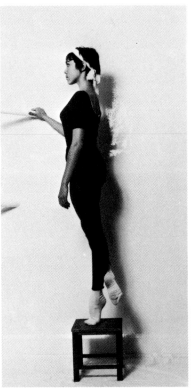

128

Patella:

1. **Chondromalacia:**

Chondromalacia patellae may be a signal for a dancer to give up. It is worth trying a spell of rest in a splint and treatment by short wave diathermy.

2. **Dislocation:**

The quicker the patella is reduced from lateral dislocation the better. It can be done by gently pressing the lateral border of the patella as the knee is extended. We have had only two cases in the Royal Ballet Company in fourteen years and both have made 100% recovery and are now ballerinas. After three to six weeks splinting, with faradism to the quadriceps, straight leg raising, and ultrasound to the medial patella ligaments, careful rehabilitation is important. (See page 82 for weight-bearing exercises.) Before starting ballet, where even barre exercises put a big strain on the recently damaged structures, the knee muscles should be fairly strong.

3. **Pain at the lower pole of the patella:**

This is a very common trouble and ultrasound is usually the most helpful treatment. There seem to be three main causes of this problem:
  (a) Working with the line of weight through the heels instead of the balls of the feet; always check this (see page 22) because, if the weight is falling behind the knee, there is much more strain on the infra-patellar ligament.
  (b) An uneven pull of the patellar ligament on the lower end of the patella caused by turning the foot out beyond the knee.
  (c) Excessive kneeling on hard floors. The soft tissue covering the lower pole becomes bruised with kneeling and the soreness then causes pain with all knee movements. This usually happens when a lot of repetition of kneeling is required of a dancer, as when rehearsing a new ballet; it is advisable to use knee-pads except for the performance.

4. **Upper border of the patella:**

Sometimes a few quadriceps fibres are strained or torn as they insert into the upper border of the patella. This is more likely to happen with an older dancer or when a dancer with stiff quadriceps is asked to do a lot of full knee bending. The treatment is short wave diathermy or ultrasound followed by straight leg raising and avoidance of weight-bearing knee flexion while there is pain.

Inflammation of Bursae behind Knee-joint:

1. A bursa under the semimembranosus insertion sometimes communicates with the knee joint causing a mild general effusion besides a local swelling. This will settle with rest and short wave diathermy.

2. A bursa under the medial head of gastrocnemius: sometimes it is hard to differentiate this from a muscle pull, and if there is any doubt I avoid massage and just give ultrasound.

Quadriceps and Tensor Fascia Lata:

Strains and stiffness are very effectively treated by ultrasound.

HIPS

1. Strained Hamstrings:

These muscles are unforgiving, and it is very important to restore full movement after an injury. The most common place for strain is the attachment to the ischial tuberosity, but it can also occur in the bellies or at the insertions. To ignore the injury and work on, even if this is possible, invariably results in reduced straight leg raising on the injured side. The most important treatment is to avoid weight-bearing as much as possible until full straight leg raising is restored. Even in walking, because of the function of these muscles, undue tension develops in them when they are injured, and this makes even gentle stretching impossible. Heat,

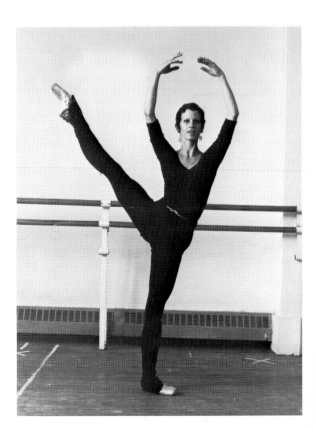

129. Note the extensive range of movement in the hip joint.

ultrasound or frictions may help, and slings in side-lying are a good way to mobilise. Certainly jumping and *arabesques* standing on the injured leg should be avoided until full range is restored.

In severe cases an X-ray examination is important in case the ischial origin has been avulsed with a fragment of bone.

Stretching the Hamstrings:

One of the best ways I know is for the dancer to lie flat and lift the injured leg with a straight knee as far as is comfortable. Resisted active hip extension is then given and as the muscles relax straight leg raising will be found to increase. The principle behind this technique can be used with any muscle group in order gently to restore a full range of passive movement.

2. Strained Adductors:

As would be expected, muscles of this group are quite often strained (Fig. 129). Sometimes the acute tenderness is on the pubic bone and sometimes in the belly of the muscle. The former should be X-rayed in severe cases because some bone may have been avulsed from the pubis. In any case rest is important until the tenderness has settled. The latter can be helped more by ultrasound and massage, and slings are very useful in restoring a full range of movement (Fig. 130).

3. Bursitis:

There are numerous bursae round the hip joint and considering the wide range of movement it is not surprising if they sometimes get inflamed. The two commonest to cause trouble are:—

    (a)   Iliopsoas bursa. This lies in front of the hip joint, between the iliopsoas

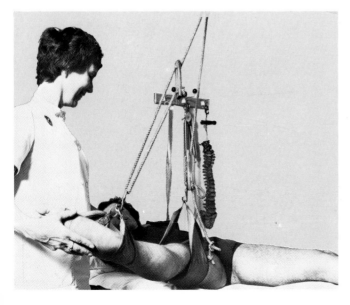

130. Slings used to mobilise after adductor or hamstring muscle strain.

tendon and the lesser trochanter. Pain is produced by active and passive flexion and internal rotation of the hip joint. Short wave diathermy and rest are the only treatments that have been found helpful.

(b)   Gluteal bursa. There is a bursa under the insertion of gluteus medius into the greater trochanter which when inflamed makes abduction very painful. If it does not settle down with ultrasound, an injection of hydrocortisone can be very effective, followed by a period of rest.

4. Synovitis or Early Arthritis:

Because there is a tendency with dancers to force all movements of the hip joints beyond their natural limits especially outward rotation, they are more prone to early wear and tear in these joints. General inflammation of the synovium is best treated with short wave diathermy and rest (Fig. 131). A more chronic symptom is limited and painful internal rotation and in this case passive mobilisation with traction will help to restore full range of movement.

THE SPINE

The very full range of movement used by dancers, and in the case of men, the continual lifting and carrying of their partners, can produce muscle and joint strains in the spine, jarring or protrusion of discs, and early degenerative arthritis.

It is very important that every joint is used to the maximum so that the strain of extreme movement is spread throughout the spine and not concentrated on one joint. Exercises for the back have been discussed on pages 18–19.

Lifting:

Strengthening exercises for the arms and shoulder girdle are an important preliminary to lifting. Press-ups can usually be done even when the dancer is off work

131. Short wave diathermy.

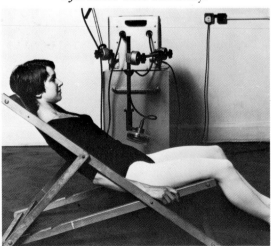

with an injury. When preparing to lift, the male dancer should stand as close to his partner as possible and bend the knees rather than lean forward at the hips. During a lift the spine should be kept as near to the normal spinal curves as possible (Figs. 20–23). Great care should be taken not to extend the back at the thoraco-lumbar junction (Fig. 90).

Diagnosis of back troubles is often difficult, but with dancers it can be further complicated because of the very full range of movement and their ability to splint a damaged joint with their own muscles, while moving above and below it, which can often be deceptive.

An X-ray is definitely recommended if the pain is severe or recurs. We have come across two cases of lumbo-sacral fusion and one of 5–6th cervical fusion. This tends to put a strain above or below the joint, and once the dancer accepts this limitation, she will stop trying to force too much movement in this area.

Because the majority of injuries with dancers are in the muscles I tend to examine them in a non-weight-bearing position. A routine examination for pain in the neck is described below:—

1. Sit at the end of a plinth with a pillow on your knee.
2. Lay the dancer on her back with her shoulders at the edge of the plinth and her head on the pillow. She should keep one hand on her abdomen and lift a finger if she gets any pain.
3. Palpate the spines of the cervical vertebrae and the muscles either side to see if there is local tenderness. If there is no tenderness on the vertebrae a muscle injury is most likely although tenderness may be caused by a strain of the muscle fibres where they are attached to bone.
4. Give gentle straight traction to the cervical spine in various positions and note whether this gives relief or pain.
5. Give assisted active neck movements supporting the weight of the head and note the painless range (Fig. 132).
6. Resist each muscle group in turn, followed by a gentle passive movement

132. Examination of neck injury.

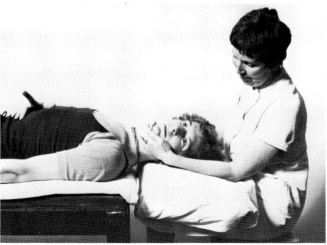

in the opposite direction. If the range of movement is greater than that obtained in 5, the limited movement is due to muscle spasm and not a block in the joint. Note also whether any active resisted movement causes pain.

7. If during 6 manipulation there is no increase in range there is either very acute muscle spasm or a joint disorder. If the latter is suspected repeat 6 but give traction during the passive movement to see if this increases the range of movement.

After this examination, combined with the history I hope to have decided whether the injury is a muscle tear, ligament strain or joint disorder.

In the same way when examining the thoracic and lumbar areas of the spine I tend to start with the dancer lying prone and see if there is any tenderness on palpating the spinous processes in the relevant area and the muscle groups either side of the spine. In the thoracic area it is also worth palpating the angles of the ribs to see if this causes pain. I then first test movement in the spine with the dancer prone kneeling. These two examinations give one a good idea of the type of injury one is dealing with before proceeding to further tests as necessary.

Muscle Strain or Tear:

These are by far the commonest injuries, which is not surprising, considering the demands of music, complicated movements and lifting. Very often the injury will not be felt while working but, as the dancer cools down, the muscles will seize up. A careful history is important because even examination of muscle tear will increase the muscle spasm. If seen immediately, the less done the better; possibly mild ultrasound, support in the form of a sorbo collar or corset, codeine and bed rest is the best treatment until the severity of the injury can be assessed. A muscle tear usually takes ten days to settle. Whether complete rest is necessary, or whether limited work can be done before then with support, depends on the severity of the injury.

Ligament Damage:

Sometimes a ligament can become overstretched either in lifting, or in an excessive movement, but because it is a relatively non-vascular structure, the pain may not be disabling until after a night's sleep, when some quite simple activity may excite it. If the strain is in a weight-bearing ligament it will give trouble for at least six weeks.

Subluxation of posterior facets:

Again the history gives a clue to diagnosis. Pain and restriction of certain movements come on fairly suddenly. Commonest in the neck, pain is often referred to the upper trapezius and there is definite block in certain movements. If this is suspected, it is well worth gently manipulating the neck. I find that by first resisting a movement, and then, as the muscles relax, moving the neck in the opposite direction with traction will often produce the wanted "click", and after that full range of movement is restored fairly dramatically. If there is much pain and spasm, treatment can be preceded by ultrasound and heat. As neither a small subluxation nor a slipped disc will show on an X-ray, it is impossible to be certain of a diagnosis. However, I have found that the dancers who present the above symptoms do not have recurring trouble which one would expect if the cause was a slipped disc.

Disc lesions:

Disc injury causing a sudden block in the joint when doing a simple movement is comparatively rare amongst young dancers. There are only two or three dancers in the Royal Ballet Company who fall into this category, and these have had less frequent recurrence since rest and sometimes traction has been used instead of manipulation. Presumably this is because, with this highly mobile group of people, the less passive disturbance there is to the joint, the better.

The bulging disc:

This is more common in men who have had to lift a lot in flexion; the symptom of pain in the back with neck flexion denotes traction on the dura and should be treated with great respect. The dancer should lie flat till this symptom has settled and then wear a corset to limit forward flexion of the spine for six weeks.

Lumbo-sacral joint:

This is a very common place for trouble because of the severe extension strain put on the joint. It is aggravated if one leg is longer than the other or if there is limited hip extension on one or both sides. Hip extension is normally much increased in a dancer from 15°–20° to sometimes as much as 50° (Fig. 133).

133. Increased hip extension.

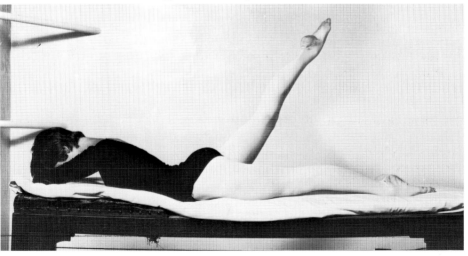

Treatment:

Although with aches and pains at the bottom of the spine a dancer will tend to think a manipulation will be the answer, this has not proved the most satisfactory treatment. As with jarring of discs from over-use at any level in the spine, the best and most lasting treatment is a spell with the weight off the spine, ideally until the non-weight-bearing range is full. Manual traction can sometimes relieve pain at the lumbo-sacral joint. This can be applied through one hip joint as follows:— With the dancer lying down the therapist cups her hands behind one knee and leans back, letting the traction pull through the hip joint to the back (Fig. 134).

Or manual traction can be given through both hip joints. In this case the dancer lies on her back with three pillows under her thighs. Padded cuffs are strapped round her ankles and these are attached to a wooden bar. The therapist then stands on a chair at the bottom of the plinth and leans back holding the bar and giving traction through the flexed hips to the low back (Fig. 135). The advantage of this method is that with the hips flexed, the lumbar spine is flat and not arched. Counter traction can be given by another therapist holding the dancer's waist. Traction is maintained for a minute or two and then released slowly. This is repeated several times.

General Back Strain in lumbar area:

This can occur in a young dancer, especially one with a mobile lumbar spine. All movements are limited and painful in extreme range and there is general aching. This is one of the few times when we have used plaster of Paris in the form of a corset to immobilise the lumbar spine for 2–3 weeks and it has been extremely successful in settling the pain and spasm.

134. Manual lumbar traction.

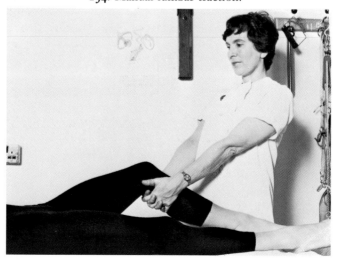

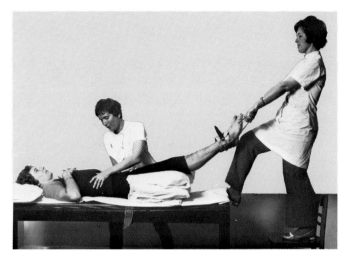

135. Manual lumbar traction through both hip joints.

SHOULDER:

1. Supraspinatus syndrome:

This produces a painful arc in abduction and is more common in men who have done much overhead lifting. Hydrocortisone injection, short wave diathermy or ultrasound are the treatments used, but a spell off lifting is important.

2. Over-developed upper trapezius:

Sometimes because of the set of the shoulders the strain of abduction is taken by the upper part of the trapezius muscles which become over-developed and constantly tense, in spite of efforts to relax them. It may be possible to relieve this by teaching the dancer to abduct the shoulder with the joint slightly more out-wardly rotated, and then compensate for the alteration in line of the arm by pro-nating the forearm.

3. Strained acromio-clavicular ligament:

Usually this is not more than a strain or partial tear amongst men who have done much overhead lifting. Ultrasound and tractions are helpful treatments and a spell off lifting.

RIBS:

Strain of the ligaments around the posterior rib attachment is not uncommon. With the dancer prone, tenderness is found at the angle of the rib rather than the spinous process. Heat and ultrasound reduce muscle spasm, and extreme upper trunk and shoulder movements should be avoided.

Glossary—Ballet Terms

A la seconde	See Fig. 10.
Arabesque	See Figs. 13, 14, 15.
Attitude	See Figs. 16, 17.
Barre	A horizontal wooden bar attached to the wall of a room about 3 feet (nearly 1m) above the ground.
Croisé	See Fig. 9.
Demi plié	Standing on both legs bending the knees without lifting the heels (Fig. 6).
Développé	A controlled unfolding of the working leg, to a finished position.
Ecarté	See Figs. 11, 12.
Effacé	See Fig. 8.
Fondu	Standing on one leg bending the knee but keeping the the heel on the ground.
Full plié	Full knee bend with heels lifted (Fig. 6).
Full point	Standing on the tips of the toes (Figs. 16, 18, 19).
Half point	Standing on the toes (ball of foot) (Fig. 17).
Pirouette	Turning on one foot.
Point Work	Dancing on the tip of the toes in specially reinforced (blocked) shoes (Fig. 18).
Port de bras	Any balletic movement of the arms.
Retiré	See Fig. 7.
Turn Out	Outward rotation of the hip joint.

Glossary—Medical Terms

Back Extension	Bending backwards (Fig. 108).
Back Flexion	Bending forwards (Fig. 109).
Bursitis	Inflammation of a bursa. There is a considerable number of bursae in the body which consist of a synovial sac and should contain only a film of fluid. When inflamed the amount of fluid increases.
Diaphragm	The sheet of muscle which separates the chest from the abdomen.
Dorsi-flexion	Pulling up the foot towards the shin.
Faradism	A small induced electric current which stimulates muscles to contract (Fig. 115).
Hamstrings	Large muscles at the back of the thigh, which bend the knee and extend the hip.
Ischial Tuberosities	The pelvic bones on which you sit and from which the hamstring muscles mainly originate.
Lumbo-sacral Joint	The joint between the bottom lumbar vertebra and the sacrum.
Malleolus.	The bony lump found either side of the ankle joint.
Non-weight-bearing Exercises	Exercise without the body weight.
Patella	Small bone (knee-cap) in front of the knee joint. Page 83.
Periostitis	Inflammation at the surface of the bone.
Plantar-flexion	Pointing the foot (Fig. 64).

Quadriceps	Large muscles on the front of the thigh, which straighten the knee.
Scoliosis	A sideways curve in the spine (Fig. 86).
Short wave Diathermy	A deep heat which can penetrate tissue (Fig. 131).
Straight Leg Raising	Lifting one leg with a straight knee (Fig. 82).
Synovitis	Inflammation of the synovial lining of a joint.
Tendinitis	Inflammation of a tendon.
Teno-synovitis	Inflammation of the sheath around a tendon.
Ultrasound	A sound wave with a frequency beyond the limit of human hearing which can penetrate up to 2 inches (5cm) under the skin causing a vibration of cells like a micromassage. This is very useful in dispersing swelling and bruising and freeing adhesions (Fig. 120).
Weight-bearing Exercises	Exercises involving the body weight.

Summary

The most important aim in treating a dancer's injuries is to restore full movement. No dancer wants to be off but complete rest is often the quickest way to recovery. The old adage "more haste less speed" is particularly relevant especially if the dancer is fairly young. This is because dancing with an injury invariably produces strain in another part of the body and, if the injury becomes chronic, it takes longer to cure and tends to leave a weak place in the dancer's body. For an older dancer the problems are different because muscle strength to support the joints becomes progressively more important year by year. It may be better to keep working carefully through an injury, provided technique is watched.

The importance of careful diagnosis and clear instructions for the road to recovery have already been stressed. It is easier to be precise with a major injury than with one which is ill defined, when both treatment and future planning are a matter of individual judgement and experience, but from the psychological point of view definite instructions are almost as important.

To recapitulate on the principles of treatment:
1. Muscle tears: Ice. Rest. Later heat and non-weight-bearing exercises till full range is restored.
2. Synovitis: Ice. Rest. Firm support in elevation. Later short wave diathermy.
3. Periostitis: Rest.
4. Ligament Strain: Ultrasound. Frictions. Support.
5. Tendonitis or Tenosynovitis: Rest. Possibly ultrasound.
6. Bursitis: Rest. Ultrasound. Hydrocortisone injection.

Before ending this book, I might add that, in spite of all the discussion and emphasis on the perfect physique, nothing is so important as the will to dance of the true artist of movement. Very often the greatest artists have to battle with considerable physical problems, while the dancer with a near-perfect physique does not have the will to persevere.

Index

Abdominal muscles, exercise 60, 61
Achilles tendon 52, 77
  peritendinitis of 80
  ruptured 79
Acromic-clavicular ligament 91
Adductors, strained 85
A la seconde 6
Anatomy 13–19
Ankle, exercise 61
  sprained 47
Ankle joint 22, 46, 74
  over-mobile 47
  sprain 73
Anklet support 48
Arabesque 17, 18, 54, 85
  epaulé 8
  1st 7, 68
  2nd 68
Arabesque penchée 8
Arch of foot 46–47
Arthritis 71
  early 86
Articular cartilage 13
Artistic temperament 65
Attitude croisé 71
  on half point 9
Attitude effacé on point 9

Back, exercise 62
  lower, exercise 59
  upper, exercise 58
Back flexion 19
Back strain in lumbar area 90
Back troubles 48
  diagnosis 87
Ball and socket joint 14
Bathing, contrast 67

Big-toe joint 42, 70, 71
  prevention of stiffness in 45
Breathing, apical 31
  diaphragmatic or abdominal 32
  exercises 31–2
  lateral 32
Bulging disc 89
Bunion 46, 68
Bursa 77
  inflammation of 83
Bursitis 85

Calf muscles 78
Cartilage, articular 13
Cervical or neck region 17
Chart, dancer's 68
Chondromalacia patellae 83
Coccyx 15
Coronary ligament 81
Croisé devant 5

Dancer's heel 76
Demi plié 4, 42
Diaphragm, over-developed 32
Diet 55
Disc injury 89
Discs, intervertebral 15
Dislocation 83
Dowell, Anthony 1
Dropped metatarsal heads 70

Ecarté derrière 7
Ecarté devant 6
Effacé devant 5
Epaulé arabesque 8
Eversion exercises 72
Exercises, abdominal muscles 60, 61

ankle 61
back 58, 59, 62
breathing 31–2
eversion 72
hip 59, 61, 62
knees 61
lifting 86
non-weight bearing 58–63, 73
quadriceps 81
spine extension 18–19
thighs 62
Extensor retinaculum 75

Faradism 70
Fatigue 52
Fibula 78
5th position 3, 10
First aid 54
1st position 2, 10
Flat foot 38
Flexor digitorum longus tendon 74
Flexor hallucis longus tendon 74
Fluid intake 56
Fondu 42, 75, 78, 80
Fonteyn, Dame Margot 29
Foot 38
    arch of 46–7
    flat 38
    injuries 68
4th position 3
Frog position 38
Full plié 4

Gable, Christopher 71
General health 55–6
Gliding joints 14
Gluteal bursa 86
Grand battement 54

Half point 71
    rise to 44
Hallux rigidus 71
Hallux valgus 68
Hamstring muscles 19, 48
    strained 84
    stretching 85
Hamstring stretch 34
Head, correct holding 24
Health 55–6
Heel 76
High arch 46
Hinge joint 14
Hip extension 89
Hip joints 17, 90
    rotary movement in 40
Hips 84
    exercise 59, 61, 62

turn-out 38
Hydrocortisone 81, 91

Iliopsoas bursa 85
Injuries and strains 52–4, 64–5, 89, 95
    and physique 65
    assessment of 66
Intervertebral discs 15

Jack-knife 19
Joints 13
    ankle 22, 46, 74
        over-mobile 47
        sprain 73
    ball and socket 14
    big-toe 42, 45, 70, 71
    gliding 14
    hinge 14
    hip 17, 90
        rotary movement in 40
    knee 34, 81, 83
    lumbo-sacral 18, 20, 50, 89, 90
    movement of 14, 16
    sacro-iliac 18
    spinal 50
    tarso-metatarsal 72

Keller's operation 71
Knee joint 34, 81
    inflammation of bursae behind 83
Knees, bruising 52
    exercise 61
    sway-back 34

Leg, lower 77
Leg length 48, 50
Leg raising 48
Lifting 10, 52
    exercises 86
Ligaments 13, 14, 48
    acromio-clavicular 91
    coronory 81
    damaged 88
    medial 81
    of ankle joint 73
    of tarsal bones 73
    strained 81, 91
    stretched 33, 38, 72
Lower back, exercise 59
Lower-leg rotation 37
Lumbar region 18
Lumbar traction 90
Lumbo sacral joint 18, 20, 50, 89, 90

Macleary, Donald 68
McMurray's click 81
Manipulation 50, 90

Medial ligament 81
Meniscectomy 81
Meniscus, torn 81
Metatarsal, fracture of base of 5th 72
  stress fracture of 70
Metatarsal heads, dropped 70
Muscle tone 27–8
Muscles 13, 14, 52
  abdominal, exercise 60, 61
  calf 78
  hamstring 19, 48, 84, 85
  strain or tear 88
  tear in belly of 79
  thigh 40
  trapezius 91
Musculo-tendinous junction 79

Neck injury 87
Non-weight-bearing exercises 58-63, 73

On point in 1st and 5th position 10
Os trigonum 77

Park, Merle 1
Patella 83
Pelvic tilt, over-correction 22
Pelvis 18
  control of 20
Peroneus brevis 72
Physique 33–51
  and injury proneness 65
  perfect 33
  problems in 33
Pliés 52, 80
Poking head 24
Positions 1–12
  1st 2, 10
  2nd 2
  4th 3
  5th 3, 10
Posterior facets, subluxation of 88
Posture 20–6
  and spinal curves 15
  correction 21, 22, 69
  faulty 20
Principal positions 1–12

Quadriceps 84
  exercises 81

Relaxation 29–30
  practising the art of 29
Retiré 4
Ribs 91
Royal Ballet Company 27, 33, 50, 64, 67, 81, 83

Sacro-iliac joints 18
Sacrum 18
Salt 56

Scoliosis 50–1
2nd position 2
Shoes 45, 54, 71
Shoulder 91
Sibley, Antoinette 68
Skeleton 12, 13
Smoking 56
Spinal joints, pains in 50
Spine 14, 86
  bottom joint of 50
  exercise to encourage extension 18–19
  flexibility of 16
  flexion of 19
  movement in 16, 17
  natural curves 15
  sideways curve in 50–1
  thoracic, rotation of 17–18
Strains. See Injuries and strains
Sublaxation of posterior facets 88
Supraspinatus syndrome 91
Sway-back knees 34
Synovitis 86

Talo-calcaneal joint 76
Tarsal bones, ligaments of 73
Tarso-metatarsal joint 72
Tendinitis 80
Tendons 74, 80
  see also Achilles tendon
Tendu 42
Tensor fascia lata 84
Thigh muscles 40
Thighs, exercise 62
Thoracic or chest region 17
Thoracic spine, rotation of 17–18
Tibia, medial border of 78
  stress fracture of 77
Tibialis anterior 78
  strained insertion 74
Tibialis posterior, strained insertion 74
  tenosynovitis or tendinitis of 74
Toes, movement of 42
Transference of weight 22
Trapezius muscles 91
Treatment 64–91, 95
  equipment 67
  home 67
  medical and surgical supplies 67

Ultrasound 73–84, 91
Upper back, exercise 58

Vertebrae 14
Vitamins 55

Water intake 56
Weight, transference of 22
Weight problems 55

X-rays 71, 73, 77, 78, 85, 87, 89